AN UNCOMMON FAITH

The Story of Missionary Jan Moses and Her Journey with Cancer

Mark Moses

This book is lovingly dedicated to Jan.
May her testimony continue to point
others to the Lord, Jesus Christ.

APPRECIATION

The feet of our faith rest on the shoulders of those
whose walk with the Lord carry us onward. The
following authors have helped me develop
a Biblical understanding of suffering.

John Piper – Desiring God
Bill Gothard – Basic Seminar
C. S. Lewis – The Problem of Pain
D. A. Carson – How Long, O Lord ?
Philip Yancy – Disappointment with God
Bruce Wilkinson – The Life God Rewards
James Dobson – When God Doesn't Make Sense

For additional copies, go to
janmoses.atspace.com

CONTENTS

Introduction..1
(February 8, 2007)

Chapter 1: A LIFE WELL LIVED..4
Early Years / Growing Spiritually / Jan and Mark /
Missionary Mom / Fruitful Years of Ministry

Chapter 2: OUR CANCER ADVENTURE BEGINS..........16
(January to April 2004)
Going to Houston / Bad News /
More Bad News / Leaving

Chapter 3: RECOVERING...30
(May to December 2004)
Together Again / An Eventful Summer /
Waiting / Returning to the Philippines

Chapter 4: THE CANCER RETURNS............................45
(January to May 2005)
Getting Settled / Work & Play / Not Feeling Well /
Leaving Once Again / Always an Encourager

Chapter 5: JAN IMPROVES..62
(June to September 2005)
Our New Home / First Website Entries /
Some Glorious Days / A Dude Ranch & Mountains

Chapter 6: A CHALLENGING AUTUMN......................82
(October to December 2005)
The Clinical Trial / Arm Fracture / Surgery /
Much to Give Thanks For / 20 Years of Service

Chapter 7: AN EMOTIONAL ROLLERCOASTER..........104
(January to April 2006)
Another House / Adjusting / In the Bones /
Leg Surgery / Recovering

Chapter 8: STILL A MOM...............................126
(May to September 2006)
Summer Activities / Adventure in D.C. /
Decisions / Out of the Trial

Chapter 9: A GROWING FAITH....................147
(October to December 2006)
Refined by Cancer / God Will Make a Way /
The Secret to Jan's Faith / Humor / Family Times

Chapter 10: "I'VE BEEN READY FOR A LONG TIME".......171
(January 2007)
Brain Surgery / Cautious Optimism / Fatal News /
Another Hemorrhage / Back to Texas

Chapter 11: JAN'S PROMOTION...................193
(FEBRUARY 2007)
No Improvement / Transfer to Hospice /
Final Days / Jan's Homegoing

Chapter 12: HER TESTIMONY CONTINUES..............208
Burial and Memorial Service / Words of Hope /
Words of Affirmation / Words of Life

Appendix 1: God and Cancer.....................228

Appendix 2: A Faith Like Theirs is Hard to Fathom....233
by Steve Blow

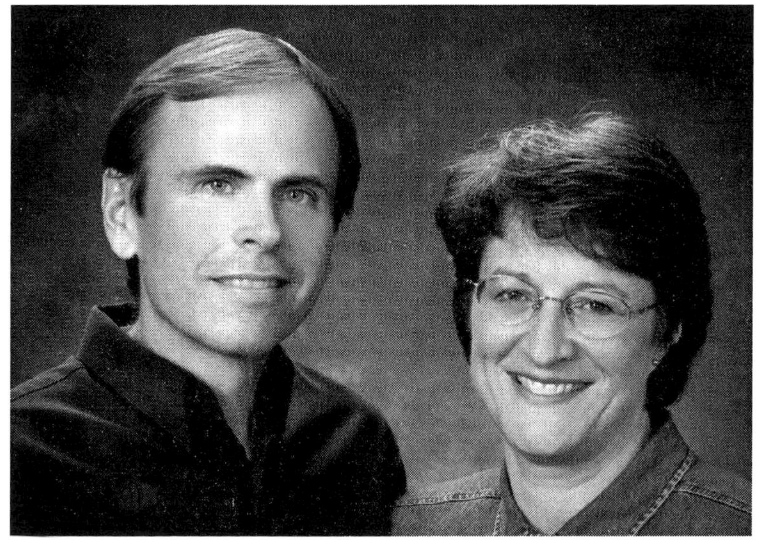

Mark and Jan - July, 2004

INTRODUCTION

"It won't be long now," the hospice nurse gravely announced. For several hours, Jan's weakening lungs had been desperately pumping air. Exhausted, her breathing had begun to slow; her fingertips turning shades of blue.

It was three years ago when our *cancer adventure* began. *"Kids, do ya'll see this odd looking spot on my arm? It's probably just some type of skin mole, but I'm going to have it taken off next week, and it could be melanoma cancer."* Jan told us then what she knew about the deadly disease, including its likely outcome. But none of us thought seriously that this could happen.

Sitting at the foot of her bed, I could feel the coldness in Jan's feet. Her hands were losing their color. At the nurse's announcement, I moved to Jan's left side, gently stroking her forehead, running my fingers through her thinned hair.

It was March 18, 2004 when we received the biopsy report: melanoma skin cancer. We were in the Philippines where melanoma is rare. After a series of calls to the States, Jan was off to MD Anderson in Houston. Thinking that the cancer was isolated, Jan would have more tissue removed, some tests done, then hopefully return soon to our ministry in the Philippines.

But while at MD Anderson, a sentinel biopsy revealed that at least one lymph node near her right arm was also infected with cancer. Standard procedure was to remove all her lymph nodes on that side, from arm to hip. Following surgery on April 21, Jan began her recovery while staying in the guest apartment of First Baptist Church of Houston. Jan's father and stepmother were there to provide food and assist Jan with her drainage tubes.

Now, Jan's father and stepmother were both near Jan's bedside, as well as Jan's brother, holding her left hand. Sara, Hannah, and Martha were on her right side, tears dampening the hurt they were feeling, watching their mother slip away. Earlier we had sung and read scripture, but now we could only whisper, *"Goodbye,"* and *"I love you."*

I couldn't help but think that it should be me in this bed instead of Jan. While Jan was recovering from her surgery in Houston, I was going about my ministry in the Philippines when, on the afternoon of April 28, 2004, I noticed blood in my urine. A CT scan later showed a large tumor sitting on top of my left kidney. I had kidney cancer.

After another series of calls to the States, the kids and I were packing and saying tearful goodbyes to a place we had called home for nineteen years. Back in Texas, my kidney was removed on May 19. A bone scan showed a 'hot spot' on my left leg, probable cancer metastasis (spread). The prognosis for stage IV kidney cancer – an aggressive cancer, was poor. Yes, it should have been me in this bed, not Jan.

It was obvious to all of us that Jan's breathing was deteriorating. The nurse now stood at the foot of the bed, stethoscope around her neck, counting the seconds on her watch. She had seen this many times before. Still, her eyes were moist. On the cabinet by the door, my cell phone rang. I waved it off. These moments were too somber, too sacred.

When we were diagnosed with our cancers, my first concern wasn't about surgeries, treatments, or emergency housing in the States for a family of 7 on a tight budget. My overriding thought during those first weeks was the question I knew everyone would be asking: Why would a loving God allow a missionary couple in the prime of their ministry, with five dependent children, to both get cancer?

Because of faithful people in our past who had taught us the Scriptures, I knew there were answers, solid answers. On May 2, 2004, I preached what I thought would be my last sermon at our little church in Iloilo City on the Philippine island of Panay. There I made my first attempts to explain why. Because of the suddenness of it all, I'm not sure anyone heard the message.

Long pauses now interrupted Jan's shallow breathing. This godly lady whose faith had impacted the lives of many, was about to enter her Savior's presence. Believing she could still hear us, we spoke words of love to her.

It would seem very odd to be thinking of blessings at such a time as this. But the past three years had brought more blessings to our family than we could have ever imagined. Thousands had prayed for us, gifts had been showered upon us, the family of God had shown their love by encouraging us every step of the way. But most of all, we had seen and experienced the presence of God; his *fingerprints* lovingly touching every day of our cancer adventure.

Jan's ministry had blossomed. Articles had been written about her faith. Her website had over thirty thousand visits. Our e-mail box was backed up with hundreds of messages of appreciation to Jan for her encouraging words. She had spoken to dozens of groups, each time her testimony was the same. God is faithful. God is good. No matter what our circumstances, we can know that God is orchestrating every event in our lives for our eternal benefit and His ultimate glory. And now Jan was about to be carried to her eternal home by the very One to whom she had given her life to serve.

It was 11 p.m. We were by her side, holding her hands, when she offered up her last breath. Her lungs emptied, her eyes closed, her race won, her spirit received, her joy made complete.

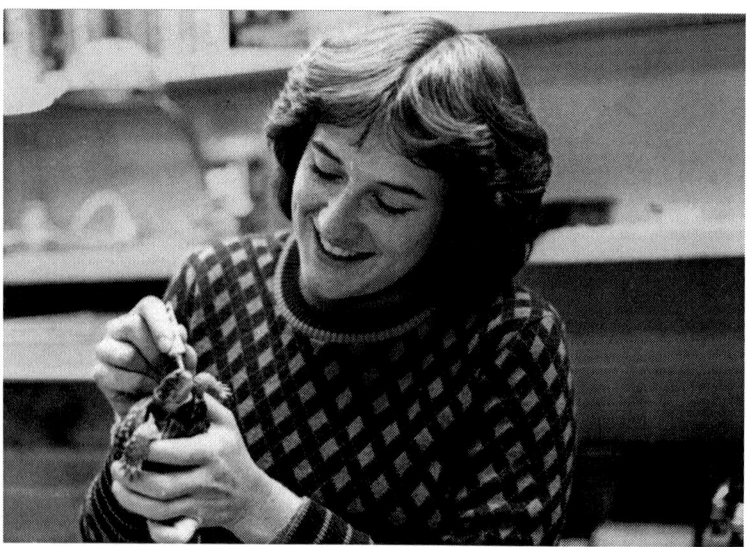

Jan, majoring in biology at the University of Virgina

Chapter 1: A LIFE WELL LIVED

Jan was alone in her dorm room. Why was she so troubled and confused? Why these feelings of emptiness and depression?

She had everything, or so it seemed. She had been the valedictorian of her high school class, voted *most likely to succeed*, honored with scholastic awards from best in math to best in science. Now at the end of her third year of college, her grade point average was nearly perfect. Everyone knew Jan, the girl with the big smile who could make friends with anyone. She had a steady boyfriend who had at least joked about getting married. With graduation just over a year away, life seemed promising for this gal who seemed to do everything right.

But everything wasn't right, and it troubled her deeply. Why all this emotional turmoil; why this inward unrest? Only later in life did Jan learn to recognize the inner workings of God's Holy Spirit, His loving efforts to strip away the fragile facades of happiness so that He could replace them with the solid anchors of truth.

Early Years

Her father was a dental student in Richmond, Virginia when Jan was born in 1956. *"I would have you know,"* Jan would later quip to her Texas friends who tagged her as a 'Yankee,' *"that I was born in the home state of Robert E. Lee and in the capitol of the Confederacy!"*

Though born on December 31, her father didn't make enough money that year to need the tax deduction. After he graduated from dental school the following year, Dr. William "Bill" Joness (two s's but still pronounced as *Jones*) moved his family to a promising practice in his hometown of Vinton, Virginia, a suburb of Roanoke. The Joness family included his wife, Betty, from California, their first born, Wynn, and now Jan. In another five years, Wayne would complete the Joness family.

Jan enjoyed the Roanoke valley, growing up within bike riding distance of the Blue Ridge Parkway. She made friends easily, but quickly became known as a "talker", a class mischief maker, and a frequent visitor to the principal's office.

"One morning we were taking a test," Jan recalled with a smile, *"and I didn't know the answer to a problem, so I rather loudly asked the girl next to me if she knew. The teacher came and tore up my paper. It wasn't the last time I got my paper tore up for talking in class. My dad was so glad when we finally got computerized report cards in the 6th grade so I wouldn't get any more bad conduct marks, like 'talks too much.'"*

Being a dentist, the Joness family lived in an upscale subdivision. Her father, a former marine, was a strict disciplinarian. TV was limited to weekends, her room had to be cleaned daily, and instant obedience to the father was mandatory. *"My dad wasn't home much,"* Jan remembered, *"but when he was home, everybody knew it. Mom was always busy in the kitchen. She was the one who tried to maintain harmony in the house.*

"My dad had a strong work ethic. Maybe it was that, plus my eagerness to learn, that helped me do so well in school. I quickly became a sponge for knowledge." With her eagerness to learn, an excellent memory, and a gregarious personality, Jan excelled in school. She got involved in track, drama, school

politics, and was even a "pom pom" girl. During her senior year, she became editor of the school newspaper. But her spiritual growth was almost non-existent.

"My family was mainly Easter and Christmas only church attenders. But one summer a friend of mine in high school invited me to a "Super Summer" camp, hosted by a popular Christian youth minister. It was there that I first heard the gospel and about what it meant to be a Christian.

"Someone there said that I needed to join a church, so I told my family that on Sunday, I was going to join the Baptist church. Not to be left out, my whole family went with me and we all joined the church that Sunday.

"I still didn't have a relationship with Jesus Christ, but I wanted to know more about Him. When I went forward with my family that Sunday morning, the minister asked if I wanted to be baptized. I thought, "Is that what this is all about?" So I got baptized, even though I wasn't saved. My dad said that this Jesus thing wouldn't last long. And he was right, it didn't."

After graduating at the top of her class, Jan was ready to leave home and be out on her own. Not knowing what to major in, Jan chose to attend the University of North Carolina at Chapel Hill. Though she only stayed a year, one incident stands out in her memory:

"A friend invited me to a chapel service. I reluctantly went. When the preacher gave an invitation, he said that after the service he wanted to shake the hand of everyone there, because he could tell by looking at their eyes whether they were truly a Christian or not. I didn't respond to the invitation and neither did I go by and shake his hand."

After one year in North Carolina, Jan decided to transfer to the University of Virginia so she could be near her boyfriend. She majored in biology, made excellent grades, had lots of friends, and an active social life. But she wasn't happy.

"I was really confused. Outwardly, I had everything the world said I should be satisfied with. But I wasn't happy. And that's where things that people had shared with me through the years began to come back and make sense. That God had created me, and He created me to be in relationship with Him. And until I was in a right relationship with Him, I would never

find satisfaction and happiness, and the joy that I have now. And so that's where I asked Christ into my life to be my Lord and Savior. And I guess that's where my priorities really changed at that point."

Growing Spiritually

"Hey Jan, why don't we have the Bible Study in your dorm room? We can post notices on the school bulletin boards."

"What," Jan responded, *"in MY room? No way, people will think I'm a fanatic!"* Jan caught herself with her words. It was her senior year. She had only been a Christian a short time and was struggling with what all it meant for her.

"Well, OK," her friend replied, *"but think about it some more."*

Jan felt relieved, but she also felt guilty. Her Savior and now her Lord, Jesus Christ, had given His life on a cross for Jan, and she was embarrassed to have a simple Bible Study in her room. Jan asked God's forgiveness and continued to attend the Bible Study, in another dorm room. She was taking her first steps as a Christian.

In May, 1979, Jan graduated with honors from the University of Virginia. God provided a wonderful job with the U.S. Fish & Wildlife Service, working on a government refuge in central Georgia. In a position similar to a park ranger, Jan lived alone in a trailer house surrounded by 35,000 acres of mixed pine and hardwood forest.

Jan fondly referred to her three years on the refuge as her wilderness experience. Like Moses in the desert, it was a maturing time for Jan as she was free to focus on her relationship with Jesus Christ. The Scriptures became precious to her.

"It was very definitely a time of growing in my walk with the Lord, because there weren't the distractions normally found in other places. It would take me 20 minutes to drive my car to church in Gray, where I was involved in discipleship groups and working with the youth. And it was an hour by bicycle to the grocery store where I could buy whole wheat bread and yogurt.

"Of course, my dad was concerned about me finding someone to marry. I told him, "Well, Dad, sometimes there are hunters here behind these trees." But I don't think that's what my dad had in mind."

Jan would often lead tours, providing information and interpretation to the visiting public. Many of these visitors were internationals. God began giving Jan a vision of ministering overseas.

"But I needed more preparation. A passage in 2 Timothy told me to "Do your best to present yourself to God, a workman correctly dividing the Word of Truth, who does not need to be ashamed, but correctly handles the Word of Truth." I felt I needed more help so I could learn to handle the Word of Truth."

So Jan set her sights on seminary. In the fall of 1982, Jan loaded up her little yellow Volkswagen with all her earthly belongings and headed to Texas.

"My friends in Georgia just knew that when I went to Southwestern Seminary in Fort Worth that I was already going into foreign missions because I was going all the way to Texas."

Jan joined Birchman Baptist Church and began her studies in earnest. Her goal was to prepare herself to be an effective missionary. Because so many of the international visitors to the wildlife refuge had been Chinese, that's where she initially focused her attention.

"Jan, you are so organized," said a friend one day who was looking in Jan's cabinet and saw a file labeled *China.* *"Why, you even have a file on your dishes!"*

"No, no," Jan corrected her, *"that's the country of China. God's calling me into missions."*

Jan and Mark

I remember that spring day in 1983 when I met Jan. As a Sunday School group leader in our church's singles department, I had planned a home fellowship. Just before arriving, I was informed that another group leader had to cancel his fellowship and that some from his group would be attending our fellowship.

I walked into the apartment. Everyone was surrounding a young lady who was teaching them the song, *I Got So Much To Be Thankful For,* and leading them with hand motions. I wondered, *"Who is this curly headed girl who can't stop smiling and jumps around like Tigger in Winnie the Pooh?"* During the greeting time, she shared about her call to missions. *"How interesting,"* I thought, because God had called me to missions, too.

During the next few weeks, we became casual friends. I would occasionally talk with her in church, or say *"Hi"* as we passed each other in the seminary hallways. During our spring break, the singles department had a weekend retreat at a nearby Christian camp. Jan and I both attended. Sometime during the second evening, I sensed God saying to me, *"Mark, she's the one!"*

I couldn't believe it. I was content on going into missions as a single. I wasn't ready for marriage. I didn't know at the time, but Jan was struggling with the same kind of thoughts. We began to do some group dating, going with others on ministry projects. I observed her character and she observed mine. Missions became the focus of our conversations.

As spring rolled into summer, we began to wonder if God might use us more effectively in missions together. Our purpose for marriage would be to glorify God and to raise children who would honor the Lord. But before I was ready to give Jan my heart, I had to first speak with her father, back in Virginia.

Jan returned home that summer to go on a bike trip with her dad, then to attend a youth camp in West Virginia with her old church from Georgia. Jan's dad had once told her that she could marry anyone, except a missionary. While on the bike trip, Jan told her dad that this missionary-to-be was interested in her.

So while Jan was away at the youth camp, this naive Texas boy flew to Virginia to meet Jan's parents. Her mother greeted me at the airport and I immediately knew where Jan got her smile. I spent three days with them, learning about

Jan and they learning about me. On the third day, Jan's father gave permission for me to marry his daughter. I met up with Jan at the youth camp, took her to a beautiful overlook at the New River Gorge outside Beckley, and proposed to her. She accepted.

We were married later that year, 1983, on her birthday, December 31. I didn't make enough money either for it to make any difference for my taxes. Jan would jokingly say that I just needed an easy way to remember our anniversary. At any rate, missions was our goal and the International Mission Board (then the Southern Baptist Foreign Mission Board) required a newlywed couple to be married at least a year before beginning the appointment process.

I finished my seminary while ministering in my home church, Birchman Baptist, as their Single Adult Minister. The church had mercy on this poor couple by allowing us to live our first year rent-free in the church's mission house. A year later we moved to an apartment across the street from our church. On August 22, 1985, David was born.

By that time we had begun the appointment process with the Mission Board. We were approved and officially appointed in December of 1985. We left for missionary orientation that spring, then left for the Philippines in May.

Missionary Mom

Jan, 2005: *"When we first got married, people would ask, "How can you bring children into this terrible world of nuclear arms, terror threats, poverty, kidnappings, and such. It may seem trite, but the song, Because He Lives, really helped answer that question for me. It says, "How sweet to hold a newborn baby... This child can face uncertain days, because He lives." And the same is true for now. My children can face uncertain days, because Christ lives. That's the sovereignty of God... Knowing He's in control... Knowing that nothing happens to us that has not passed through His protective hand of love, and that He can use for good."*

Those days of uncertainty were waiting for us as

our truck rolled into Roxas City, on the northern part of the Philippine island of Panay. It was January, 1988. We had finished a year and a half of language study in Iloilo City, on the southern side of Panay. Sara had joined our family 3 months earlier on October 9. We had just returned from the funeral of Jan's mother in Virginia, who had finished her ten year battle with breast cancer. Now we were following a flat bed truck, carrying all our belongings, into the city where we would begin our work.

We moved into an 800 square foot apartment that had no running water, no air-conditioning, no telephone, and occasional electricity. Curious neighborhood children would gather by the dozens in front of our window to watch the Americans adjust to their new home. Little David enjoyed the attention; mom and dad had a different opinion. Still, it was the place and the people to whom God had called us to serve, and He gave us the grace to live for two and a half years in that little apartment.

Our efforts failed to produce a church that first term. But we learned a great deal about the culture and sharpened our language skills. Plus, we established many friendships that were significant in our later years of ministry. My work would sometimes carry me to remote forested areas where there were no roads; where Filipinos lived simply in bamboo homes with thatched roofs. Baptisms were done in the river and Bible studies were held under coconut trees.

Jan's focus was in the home. She spent her days preparing nutritious meals, keeping David and Sara healthy, and reading to them daily. She also kept up a steady stream of correspondence to fellow missionaries and to friends back in the States. As an extrovert, Jan was challenged by living in such an isolated place away from other Americans. Our third biggest budget expense after food and rent was postage stamps. But the Lord used this isolation to motivate us toward developing many close friendships with Filipinos.

Before the end of our first term, Hannah was born on February 6, 1990. Many would comment in later years about the maturity of our children. Much of the credit goes to Jan. We decided early on that we would not have a TV in our home. Neither would we allow rock music of any sort. We didn't want the Holy Spirit to have any competition in winning the hearts of our children.

Jan was diligent to match the learning styles of each child with the best available home school curriculums. She wanted our children to be surrounded with readily available educational resources. Almost all undesignated gifts we received purchased quality books. Our little library would eventually grow to about five thousand volumes over a period of twenty years.

Jan's passion for God's Word carried over to our home schooling. By the time David was seven, Jan had led him to memorize several Psalms and the whole book of James. David, Sara, and eventually Hannah would often recite long Scripture passages as part of my birthday and Christmas presents. Cross stitched Bible verses decorated our home.

Since Jan and I were careful to choose our children's friends, many would often ask about their socialization. *"Won't they be shocked when they get out into the real world?"* But Jan would respond by saying, *"We WANT our children to be shocked by all the evil they see in the world. They ought to be shocked. Our goal is to raise children who have the maturity of character to know right from wrong, who have the courage to say "no" to the wrong and wisdom to say "yes" to the right."*

Fruitful Years of Ministry

After our furlough in 1990, we returned to Roxas City with renewed enthusiasm to share Jesus Christ and see Filipinos grow toward spiritual maturity. We opened a ministry center in the downtown area which eventually became the location of our first church. The center served as a base for evangelistic efforts, Bible studies, and discipleship training.

By this time we had moved into a house that gave us more space for home schooling, including space for our growing library. We welcomed Martha into our family on September 12, 1993. I had the joy (though I didn't see it as joy at the time) of delivering Martha because Jan chose to labor at home a bit too long.

Although we did have "helpers", it was still incredible how Jan was able to juggle her responsibilities of managing the home, planning the meals, home schooling the children, and ministering to our neighbors. For example, after celebrating Martha's first birthday, Jan decided to give Sara a special 7th birthday party. She chose the theme of 101 Dalmatians and proceeded to decorate the house with 101 doggie cutouts highlighted with streamers and hundreds of doggie footprints throughout the house.

This was also going to be an evangelistic effort. She planned and designed games that could be played at different locations around our house. With our helpers, she planned and prepared a complete meal, along with cake and other deserts. Jan then sent out invitations to our neighbors and friends.

The house was packed. Even the parents enjoyed the games and the food. After I gave a devotional, Jan and I made the rounds speaking with as many as we could. Afterwards, Jan included a gospel presentation in each of the *"Thank You"* cards she sent out to whose who attended.

Although we have many wonderful memories of our time in Roxas City, it was also a challenging time in regards to our health. During a three year period, Jan and I were sick with malaria, typhoid, dengue fever, and amoebic dysentery. Tuberculosis and hepatitis were constant threats. Despite Jan's best efforts to protect the children, all of them were eventually infected with hepatitis A.

When we returned from our 1995 furlough, a new position had opened for us in Iloilo, a larger city on the southern end of our island, the place where we had lived during language study. We said tearful goodbyes to our friends in Roxas, but were comforted by knowing they were only a two hour visit away.

After a few weeks in Iloilo, Jonathan was born on May 11, 1996. Jan was already exhausted from leaving the States and moving to Iloilo. Jonathan's post-birth hospital stay for lung infection, plus other factors, led Jan into periods of depression. Although she sought counseling, it was her daily meditation on Scripture that helped her overcome negative emotions. She gained new understanding of God's purposes for adversity, and how suffering can be one of our greatest means for spiritual growth.

As our family grew, so did the challenge of home schooling different grades at one time. Jan, being a self-confessed perfectionist, soon found herself exhausted trying to research every curriculum, prepare daily lessons, and teach every subject. In desperation one day she cried out to me, *"I just can't do it all; I give up!"*

In a rare flash of insight, I responded with these words of wisdom, *"Well honey, something is better than nothing."* I suppose if Jan were a violent woman, she would have slapped me. That's not what her hurting heart needed to hear.

Nevertheless, the words stuck. Days later, Jan acknowledged that she had been pondering on my comment and decided there was some truth to it. She even changed her philosophy of home schooling, saying that it was a huge relief to know she didn't have to do everything to perfection. Our homeschool logo became S.B.N. (Something is Better than Nothing). In the following years, Jan would regularly remind herself that she didn't have to research and teach everything, but only do what she could.

Then one day Jan realized that S.B.N could also stand for Simple Bare Necessities. You remember *The Jungle Book* song...

> *Look for the bare necessities,*
>   *the simple bare necessities,*
> *Forget about your worries and your strife.*
>   *Oh, yeah.*
> *I mean the bare necessities,*
>   *that's why a bear can rest at ease;*
> *With just the bare necessities of life.*

Well, Jan was hooked. She had SBN printed on our shirts and whenever someone would ask its meaning, the family would break out into the Simple Bare Necessities song.

Despite some difficulties with one of our largest churches, this term proved to be one of our most fruitful. We saw several churches started, as well as others experiencing growth, both numerically and spiritually. The children continued to do very well academically, socially, and spiritually. Our circle of friends and our sphere of influence grew dramatically. Through our ministries, we were seeing the Holy Spirit change lives.

Years later, Jan would reflect on our seasons of missionary service with these words, *"We're very thankful that our family grew up overseas, we've felt incredibly blessed. It's wonderful to get to this point in life, and have no regrets, and to be very thankful for the life we have lived. And that's wonderful; that is a blessing."*

These blessings continued into the beginning of our fourth term in 2001. By now Jan and I felt that we had matured as missionaries. We were seeing spiritual grandchildren, as those to whom we had ministered to were in turn impacting the lives of others. Our children were true TCK (third culture kids), having adopted many of the positive Filipino traits as their own.

But I think one of the most painful days of our lives came in 2003 when we had to say goodbye to David as he left for college. The tears just wouldn't stop flowing as David's plane left the runway. Jan took the other kids to a downtown mall for some distracting activities, while I went home and cried for nearly an hour.

A major chapter in our lives had closed. Our nest was emptying. For the first time, one of our children would be living half a world away. But a new chapter was about to open that would bring us back together.

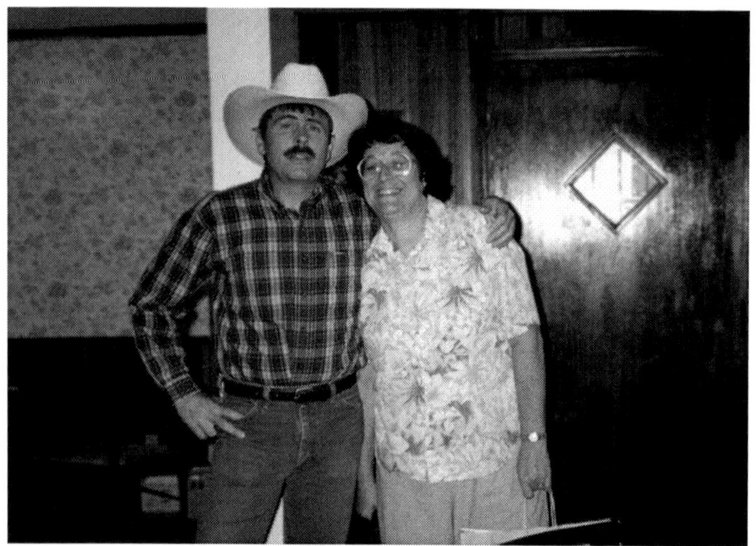

Mark and Jan ready for adventure

Chapter 2: OUR CANCER ADVENTURE BEGINS

January is my favorite month in the Philippines. The temperature is mild; the humidity low. Christmas usually leaves us feeling good. The new year brings fresh starts and renewed commitments.

But this January was unusually busy. I was buried deep in the task of translating our discipleship materials. A new church start north of Iloilo was demanding my time. Several church leaders from the First Baptist Church of Houston were coming to conduct a large evangelistic campaign that was scheduled for the fourth week of January. This added to Jan's duties, since she would be expected to feed and host the many American and Filipino visitors who would pass through our home in the weeks to come.

"I really ought to have this looked at," Jan commented one evening as she was showing me a darkened mole on her upper right arm.

"Honey, that doesn't look good. What do you think it could be?"

Jan named off a list of possibilities, including melanoma

skin cancer. *"But doctors here probably don't even know what melanoma looks like, so I'll have to wait until we're in Manila next month for Home Schoolers Meeting and have it biopsied."*

On February 19, 2004, Jan consulted with a U.S. trained dermatologist in Manila. Five days later, the mole was removed with the initial diagnosis as Superficial Basal Cell. But the dermatologist was experienced enough to request a second opinion, which required the tissue sample to be sent to the States for better analysis. On March 18, Jan received a call from the dermatologist. It was malignant melanoma.

Jan's reaction was not of shock, fear, or worry. Her mother had cancer at an early age and Jan figured she would eventually get it, too. In the days before March 18, Jan had been reminding herself that *"all the days ordained for me were written in your book, before one of them came to be"* (Psalm 139: 16). *"My times are in your hands"* (Psalm 31:15). Jan was amazingly calm, reflecting the confidence she had in her Lord and her willingness to rest in Him.

But life changed for us in a big way that day. Not that we were thinking Jan would die. The pathology report indicated a good possibility that all the cancer cells had been removed, although the findings also recommended further surgery should be done to remove more tissue. But Jan's focus changed that day from home schooling mom and missionary, to determined cancer fighter.

It's not that Jan was afraid to die; she wasn't. But she had a keen sense of responsibility to do all she could to protect and preserve the body which the Lord had given her. *"Do you not know that your body is the temple of the Holy Spirit, who is in you, whom you have received from God?"* (1 Corinthians 6:19).

On March 21, Jan wrote to our prayer supporters: *"People ask me how I am feeling... I am excited to see what God is going to do. This didn't catch God by surprise. I know God wants to use our circumstances and problems to transform us into the likeness of Jesus Christ... I don't want to miss what He has for me to learn."*

Going to Houston

The dermatologist in Manila told Jan that there was really nothing more they could do for her. Dark skinned Filipinos never got melanoma, so no one knew how to treat it. Jan would need further follow up in the States.

Jan searched the internet, made telephone calls, and decided MD Anderson in Houston would serve her needs the best. But where to stay? She remembered the evangelistic team from First Baptist Church of Houston that had come to Iloilo in January. She called. Within hours, the church's guest apartment was made available. Several members from the church volunteered to take care of her once she arrived.

I ask that you pray that I am sensitive to God's spirit during this time and that indeed I will be His witness at MD Anderson. I have heard that it is such a depressing place – as cancer can be to those who have no hope. I pray that I will be able to give hope to others that I meet during this time.

I was praising God this morning (loudly while getting ready for worship), *"My hope is in You, Lord, my strength is in You, Lord, my trust is in You, Lord – in You, it's in You."* Rejoice in the Lord always!

Jan and I decided that I would stay in Iloilo to continue my mission work, and the children would stay in the comfort of our home and continue their school work. Jan wanted to spend time with the Lord and do some more research. She knew both tasks would be difficult if she also had to take care of her family. Anyway, we expected reports to show that there was no more melanoma, and that Jan could then return to Iloilo.

On March 27, 2004, Jan shared from her journal:

Last Sunday we read Psalm 121 in worship and I felt that this was God's word for me during this time...

1. *I will lift up my eyes to the mountains; from whence shall my help come?*
2. **My help comes from the Lord**, *who made heaven and earth.* (And made me, too!)

3. *He will not allow your foot to slip; He who keeps you will not slumber.* (I may be sleeping on this side of the world while you all are awake and vice versa -- but God isn't sleeping any of that time.)
4. *Behold, He who keeps Israel will neither slumber not sleep.*
5. *The Lord is your keeper; the Lord is your shade on your* **right hand**. (I have been diligent since coming to the Philippines to wear sunscreen, carry my umbrella and other precautions. But from now on, I'm claiming the Lord as my shade. And yes, the cancer is on my right arm.)
6. **The sun will not smite you by day**, *nor the moon by night.* (SMITE - Hebrew "nakah", which means to kill, strike down, destroy, defeat. The NIV says "to harm" but to smite is more serious than that. I have been harmed by the sun but I am claiming God's word that I will not be destroyed by it.)
7. *The Lord will protect you from all evil;* **He will keep your soul**. (Jesus said don't be afraid of what can destroy your body but what can destroy your soul. No matter what happens to this body, God will keep my soul -- that part of me that will live with Him in eternity.)
8. *The Lord will guard* **your going out and your coming in** *from this time forth and forever.* (God knows all about my travels!)

We said goodbye to her at the airport, confident she would be back in a few weeks at the most. To save time and money, Jan scheduled her preliminary blood work and scans to be done in Manila, on her way out of the country. She arrived in Houston on April 1, with her father and step-mother joining her a couple of days later.

In her April 7, 2004 prayer letter, Jan said:

I am getting to experience many new adventures -- photo ID bracelet, digital x-ray, automatic paper towel dispenser. When this week is finished, I will have had 3 radioactive injections (I wonder if I glow in the dark! As I have gone from lab to x-ray to scan to surgeons to anesthesiologists, I have thought about my mom as she faced her first cancer surgery when she was only 45 years old. And yet I have gone with such a sense of joy and peace that only comes from the grace of God.

While I was 'frettin' this morning about the delay, and thinking of all that I needed to DO at home in the Philippines, God reminded that this was a time He had given me...to sit at His feet and be a Mary. A time of retreat -- which I so often wish for in the busyness of home. How could I have not seen this opportunity! I was able to spend some quality time in the Word this morning and can rejoice now that He has given me this time. So He has brought me back to a place of contentment and resting in Him and in His timing.

"I cry out to God most High, to God, who fulfills his purpose for me... My heart is steadfast. .. I will sing and make music" (Psalm 57).

"Bad News"

Back in Iloilo, the children went about their school work. I continued with the translations and preparing for our semi-annual Associational Meeting the third week of April. We were calm, until Jan called on April 10. A routine procedural surgery revealed one sentinel lymph node was positive for melanoma. Jan's cancer had spread beyond her arm. This was our worst fear. There was now a likely possibility that the cancer had begun metastasizing (spreading) to other parts of her body. I sent out a prayer letter:

Well, here's an e-mail I wish I didn't have to write. Jan called this morning with the pathology results of her lymph node biopsy. Of the two that were removed, one tested positive for melanoma and the other was unclear, requiring further examination. During the next few days, she will have a more thorough CAT scan and an MRI. Next week, probably on the 22nd, they will remove the other 17 to 20 lymph nodes under her right arm.

As for what this means for us, we don't know yet... Though we may not understand God's ways and timing at this point, I've learned long ago that I don't have to understand in order to have complete faith and trust in Him. So we press on with much appreciation for your prayers and concern.

Back in Houston, doctors were scheduling Jan for pre-operative tests, including a CT scan of her chest and a MRI scan of her brain. Jan was upbeat:

After telling a friend that I was staying in Houston longer than I anticipated because I found the traffic thrilling, she told me I needed my head examined. I told her not to worry -- they were doing that on Friday!"

I know that your prayers are sustaining me while I am here and Mark and the children in Iloilo. I was not surprised by last week's report -- I felt that God had been preparing me. One passage that He led me to last weekend was Psalm 112 -- *"Even in darkness, light dawns for the righteous. Surely he will never be shaken... He will have no fear of bad news; his heart is steadfast, trusting in the LORD."*

So when the physician called and said, *"I've got bad news: the cancer is in the lymph nodes."* I said, *"You know, I'm not surprised. And God is not surprised."* You know, bad news doesn't have to rattle me. I know God is sovereign; He is in control."

I know it is God's grace that is sustaining me. I feel like I am on a hydrofoil (these are our "fast boats" in the Philippines that ferry us between islands). A hydrofoil rides on a cushion of air over the water. You may feel motion but you are not jerked and bumped about like on a regular boat. God is that cushion of air, keeping me above the rough waves. (For you pastors, that may not be very theological, but that's how I feel!) What a joy to sing in worship this morning: *"I know not why God's saving grace to me He hath made known. Nor why, unworthy, Christ in love redeemed me for His own. But I know whom I have believed and am persuaded that He is able to keep that which I've committed unto Him against that day"* (2 Timothy 1:12).

More "bad news" followed in a few days. The CT scan on April 16, 2004, showed suspicious nodules in both of Jan's lungs, possible cancerous metastatic (spread) melanoma. I wrote again:

Thank you for your continued prayers for Jan. The results of her CT scan were not encouraging. While the MRI scan was negative, the CT scan found several suspicious places on her lungs. The largest one is 4 mm and the others are 2 - 3 mm. The scan cannot diagnose melanoma, it merely reveals abnormalities. Jan is working to get a Tuberculosis test so we can explore that as a possible reason for the abnormalities. Still, we know it could be the melanoma.

She will have her remaining lymph nodes under her right arm removed on Thursday, the 22nd. It is an extensive surgery that will require at least one month recovery. Her dad and step-mom are there with her. The doctors will reexamine the lungs in a few weeks to see if there is any change. While these developments seem to increase the likelihood that we will need to return to the U.S. soon, there is still a chance that Jan could return here if she recovers well from the surgery and the suspicious areas on her lungs do not grow.

Jan is well aware of what she is facing, yet she remains confident that the Lord has a perfect plan for all of this, regardless of the outcome. The children and I continue to plod along in our work. Jonathan has his 8th birthday on May 11. I had to explain to him today that mom would not be able to make it back by then. He said it will be OK as long as he gets his carrot cake and ice-cream. I know the Lord will give us the grace we need when we need it. As I told Sara and Hannah, God knew before Jan was ever born that this was going to happen. What a comfort to know He is walking beside us each step of the way.

On April 21, twenty-seven lymph nodes were surgically scraped from Jan's right side, none of which were positive for melanoma. Jan's father and step-mother took care of her. The daily care of her drainage tubes was tedious and cumbersome.

Still, a week into her recovery, she typed out a prayer letter, using her left arm:

> Greetings! Like the demoniac in the book of Mark, I am fully clothed and in my right mind. (Well as far as me being in my right mind, that has been debatable for some time! At least I did take a bath and have clean clothes on!)
>
> I am feeling really great, both in my body and spirit. Yes, there is post-op pain as to be expected but I think I am doing really good. I put some praise music on the CD player and am trying to walk around the apartment for 15 minutes, twice a day.   I even kicked my legs up a few times! In reading a book Fighting Cancer, that was given to me at MD Anderson, there have been SCIENTIFIC double blind studies that show that people who are prayed for recover faster from surgery and have fewer side effects. This is a SECULAR book. Wow! No wonder I am feeling SO GREAT -- the best I have felt in a long time! Thank you so much for your many prayers.
>
> We are still in a waiting mode until the results are back on these lymph nodes; then the team here in the melanoma clinic will work up a treatment plan and we should know more about what life will hold in the coming months. I am hoping that we will know something by the end of the first week in May but one thing I have learned these past few weeks is to put my hope in God alone -- and not getting my expectations up that I will know something any sooner than His time frame.
>
> I am confident that He is working good in all of this -- in my life, in my family, in our people group in the Philippines. I know that He is perfectly able to wipe out every cancer cell. But like Shadrach, Meschach and Abednego said in Daniel when threatened with the fiery furnace: *"The God we serve IS able to save us but even if he does not..."* That doesn't change my faith. My faith is based on God's character -- not circumstances or what we can see and feel. What do I know about God? Psalm 145 (the Psalms are a great place to camp in times like this) says that God is good, righteous, gracious, compassionate, slow to anger, rich

in love, faithful, near to all who call -- and He gives food at the proper time (i.e. information that is needed at the proper time).

I like what one pastor prayed regarding the cancer cells: Job 38: 8-11 says that when God made the seas, He said, *"This far you may come, no farther; here is where your proud waves halt."* This is my prayer for the "suspicious" lesions in my lungs -- that the cancer cells will halt and come no farther. I am praying that the repeat scan (to be done in 6 - 8 weeks) will show that these lesions are gone and we will give God the glory. But even if they are not gone, God is still to be praised, for He is a good and loving God.

Pray for Mark. He was to have had a seminar in Antique province this week, but he went to the doctor instead. I haven't heard yet what is the matter with him.

Thanks so much for your prayers. In reading through information given me, the most important element in fighting cancer is a good support group -- and I have a fantastic one! I don't think anyone has a better support than I do through my family, our mission family and the International Mission Board, and our network of Southern Baptist churches who are so faithful to pray, call, and send cards. It is fantastic and no wonder that I feel so great today! So blessed to be your missionary.

> *"Though an army* (cancer) *besiege me,*
> *my heart will not fear,*
> *Though war break out against* (within) *me,*
> *even then I will be confident.*
> *I am still confident of this:*
> *I will see the goodness of the Lord*
> *in the land of the living.*
> *Wait for the Lord; be strong and take heart*
> *and wait for the Lord"* (Psalm 27).

More Bad News

The morning of Wednesday, April 28, was hot and humid, like most days in the tropics. I traveled to one of our churches where I met with two pastors. We discussed issues that had been brought up during last week's Associational Meeting. After a quick lunch of dried fish, green vegetables, and rice, I dropped by the home of another pastor who had requested some marital counseling for him and his wife. It was late afternoon by the time I returned home.

After being gone all day, I made a straight line to the restroom. Needless to say, I was shocked as I filled the toilet with red urine.

A few minutes later, Hannah passed me in the hallway while I was flipping through our medical guide books. *"What's wrong Dad, are you sick?"*

"Well maybe," I replied, and then I shared with her about what might cause bloody urine, including the possibility of kidney cancer. It was always our policy to be up front with everyone in our family and to hold nothing back. This, along with God's grace, has helped the children adjust to our health challenges, knowing we were not hiding anything from them.

Aware of what I might be facing, I canceled my trip the following day to Antique Province where I was to speak at a youth camp. I went to a clinic and asked for a sonogram. An hour later, sitting in a nearby restaurant, I read the results: enhancing huge solid mass on left kidney. Further imaging advised.

I found another doctor who wrote me a request for a CT scan, but the scan couldn't be done until the next day. So I went home. Although there was no more blood in my urine, the Lord prepared me during my quiet time for what likely lay ahead.

The next morning, Friday, April 29, I laid on a cold, flat bed as the CT scanning machine zapped me with x-rays. Once completed, the normally jolly doctor's assistant returned with somberness in his voice. *"Don't worry,"* he said while trying to hide his emotions, *"God will take care of you."*

I knew then that I had cancer.

A few minutes later I was dressed and standing behind the radiologist (and next to a few of our concerned church members. No HIPAA laws here) as we looked at the computer screen that showed an apple sized tumor sitting on my left kidney. The church members wanted to encourage me by sharing stories of other cancer patients who had been cured. But by now I knew enough about cancer to know my prognosis.

I returned home and shared the news with the children. We discussed possible scenarios and even laughed at the oddity of having parents getting cancer at the same time. I called Jan. She wasn't quite as amused. Later, Jan would share that her initial reaction was one of anger, then awe, realizing God must be up to something really big. After talking with Jan, I withdrew to the computer and wrote the following:

Well, here's another e-mail I wish I didn't have to write. A few hours ago, I (Mark) had a CT scan and the results confirmed that I have a rather large kidney tumor. Last Wednesday I was surprised to see blood in my urine. An ultrasound on Thursday suggested a large mass on my left kidney. This morning it was confirmed. On the positive side, it appears not to have metastasized to nearby organs. Lymph nodes are normal in size. The standard procedure is to remove the infected kidney along with the attached tumor. Our medical guide, meaning to be encouraging, says, "about 7 in 10 people who have a kidney tumor removed survive more than 5 years, even if the tumor was large."

Sara, Hannah, and I have been quite amused at the timing of it all. Jan lovingly accused me of trying to race her to heaven. Actually, as long as the cancer has not spread, my long term prospects for post-surgical recovery are good. Still, I will have to make several near term decisions, such as where to have the surgery, in Iloilo or in Manila? Who will stay with the children while I'm in the hospital? Fortunately, recovery from this surgery is normally not lengthy, with the remaining kidney quickly taking on the work of the removed one.

Right now I have a tremendous peace about this new development in the health saga of our family. Just as God knew Jan would develop melanoma cancer, so God knew also, before the day I was born, that this would happen to me. God knew the day Jan and I were married that this would happen, yet he still brought us together and blessed us with a wonderful ministry here in the Philippines. And He knows exactly what is to come.

As in Jan's case, so now in mine, what I pray for is not so much for healing (although that would certainly be welcomed) but rather that God will be glorified. There are many other ways, besides healing, for God to be glorified. Perhaps God would allow a person or a couple to go through the trials of cancer in order for him/them to demonstrate a firm trust in the Lord, Jesus Christ. I believe steadfast faithfulness in the midst of greater sacrifices brings more pleasure to God's heart. *"For without faith, it is impossible to please Him"* (Hebrews 11:6).

It's not that God enjoys inflicting sickness in order to elicit more faith. (God did not author sickness; He is not to blame for this.) Rather, it is a good show of faith in the midst of adversity that allows God to joyfully bestow greater rewards for us in eternity. *"He is a rewarder of those who seek Him" (Hebrews 11:6). "For your Father has chosen gladly to give you the kingdom"* (Luke 12:32). *"...rejoice in that day and leap for joy, because great is your reward in heaven"* (Luke 6:23). God makes decisions from the basis of eternity; we too often from the basis of this temporary life. If God, from the perspective of eternity, saw that a strong show of faith for a short term would lay up greater rewards in eternity than small steps of faith in the long term, then why would I want to pray for a healing that would rob me of those eternal rewards?

Don't get me wrong. I want very much for Jan and I both to be fully healed, especially when I think of the children. But what I am saying is that God knows better than me, he sees further than I can see, He knows which road to take. I know God has my, Jan's, and our children's best interest in His heart. And He is going to make decisions that will give us the greatest measure of eternal blessings (which we don't deserve), thus giving Him the highest glory. And that's what I want.

Thank you so much for your prayers. I know it is because of this that God is pouring out His grace and peace on our family.

Leaving

I guess it was a bit naive of me to think I could pack an overnight bag, drive down to the local hospital, have them take out my cancerous kidney, and be back to work in a week. That's why I balked the next morning when our mission board personnel insisted I needed to return to the States with the children.

I cried, not because of the seriousness of my condition, but because we would need to pack and leave in a week. Leave our "home" and ministry. Leave our friends and the people to whom God had given us a heart to love, not knowing if we would ever return.

The children cried, too, for the same reasons. Listen as Hannah shares her feelings during this time in a paper she wrote called "Leaving":

> That week replays hazily in my memory, like a haunting dream that won't go away. It was May, the hottest month of the year in the Philippines. One sweaty day drifted into the next as we sorted, packed, and said our goodbyes.
>
> We were very limited in what we could bring on the airplane – two seventy pound suitcases each. So how do you pack your life into two suitcases? Do I pack the precious books I learned to read by or pack my schoolbooks? Do I bring my baby clothes or clothes I can wear now? Our photo albums filled up an entire box by themselves. We had to be very objective and strictly monitor what went in our luggage. The stress of that kind of sorting, in that amount of time, taxed our energy and drained our emotions.
>
> Then Friday came, the final day in a chapter of my life that was about to close forever. Before leaving for the airport, I purposed not to cry. But as we said goodbye to our two little dachshounds we let the tears fall. Our dachshounds looked up with their mournful large brown eyes, and whined in bewilderment as to why we were crying. We parted, wondering if we would ever see them again, and watched from the car window

as they stuck their heads between the bars of the gate to watch us drive off.

All week long I had carried a veneer of sanity knowing, though, that the slightest provocation would make me break down. The veneer barely held on the way to the airport, but began to crack when we saw the crowd at the terminal. The tears began pouring again as we said goodbye to our church members, friends, and Filipino surrogate family. *"We'll see you again,"* they whispered in encouragement. Reluctantly, we walked to the plane, and it carried us to the States.

For now my family resides in the States. I am in a different culture, a different country, a different continent, and a different world. Instead of waking up in the morning to the soothing breezes of a tropical wind, I wake up shivering because of the dry cold air. Instead of seeing other Americans twice a year, I see them every day. Instead of going to a movie on public transportation and the entire evening costing a dollar, I now ride in a private car and the movie costs ten times as much. Instead of walking across rice patties to get to a dirt floor church, we walk across a wide paved parking lot to enter a huge carpeted sanctuary. Instead of listening to a single guitar and one worship leader in a church of thirty-five members, we listen to an orchestra and a choir in a congregation of a thousand. Instead of seeing my best friends at least twice a week, I don't see them at all.

As for now, I'm learning to be an American. We ought to "bloom where we are planted," and we are all aiming to do that. I will never forget the Philippines, our friends there, or the lessons I learned there, about hospitality and how we can all do with less than what we have here in the States. And even though it was difficult and heartbreaking to leave, I would not trade my years in the Philippines for the world. They have made me who I am. For now I am in the States, and I will learn to adapt to this *foreign* culture. What happens now to my family is in God's hands.

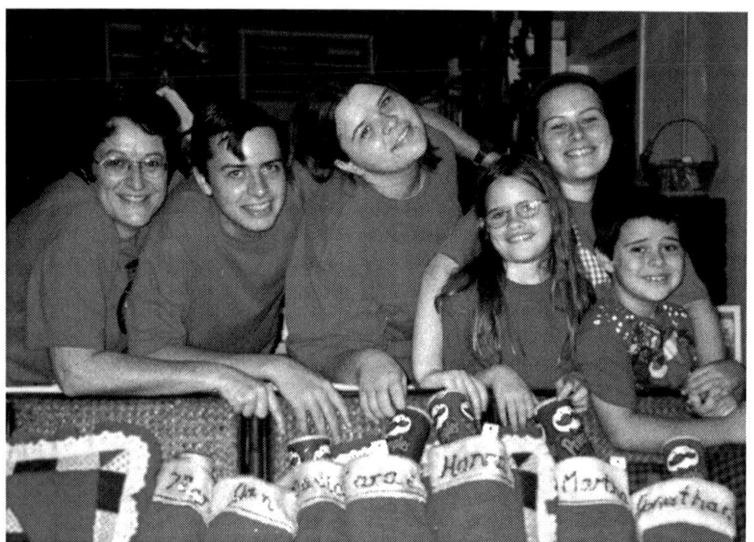
A family Christmas

Chapter 3: RECOVERING

I was alone in the backseat, gazing out the car window at the nighttime. Street lights and car lights, home fronts and store fronts, people rushing and the stars resting, it is amazing what you see when you know life is short.

Next to me was a large envelope with my medical reports of the past week: *Bone scan...abnormal uptake focal area on left femur of unknown origin...suspicious for skeletal metastatic renal cell carcinoma.* Hmmm, medical reports were always noncommittal. But my surgeon didn't want me hanging onto false hopes. That hot spot on my upper left leg bone was likely my kidney cancer, an aggressive cancer, beginning to spread throughout my body. Prognosis would be a few months, maybe a year at best.

It was May, 2004. We had been in the States for a week. All kidney surgeons at MD Anderson were attending a conference, so our mission board doctor had to schedule me with a surgeon in Dallas. A bigger problem was where to find housing for a family of 7. Church mission homes were usually booked years in advance. When our mission board office called the First Baptist Church of Dallas, they had just received a cancellation on one of their mission houses. It was available. I think the Lord did that for us.

But Jan was still in Houston, healing slowly, not yet released by her doctor for travel. In Dallas, I had blood tests done on Tuesday, the 11th, met with the surgeon on the 12th, a bone scan and a CT scan on the 13th, and received the scan results on the 14th. Later that morning we (minus David who was finishing up his college semester) drove to Houston to see Jan, whom we had been separated from for over two months.

Together Again

The joy of seeing Jan again made me forget about the growing pain in my left leg. After showing us her drainage tubes, she brought us up to date on her situation. She would likely do some type of chemotherapy after she recovered from her surgery. The spots in her lungs were especially worrisome. The surgical incision area was healing slowly. The doctor said she wasn't resting enough. Jan figured, *"Maybe my definition of rest as a home school, missionary mom of 5 in a third world country is different than his definition."* So Jan said she would have to try harder at resting. It would be a week, though, before she could travel to Dallas.

Jan was excited about a phone call she had just received from MD Anderson. One of their renal cell (kidney) specialists could probably do my surgery later next week. But I was already scheduled for surgery in Dallas on the 19th. Big decision. Jan and I decided we needed to pray.

I remember Jan and I alone in the apartment bedroom, kneeling by the bed, holding hands as I prayed, *"Lord, You know the best place for me to have this surgery. We need to hear from You. Please give us an indication, maybe a word from You through a friend, or maybe a phone call that would help us know what to do next."*

At that very moment the telephone rang. Jan and I looked up at each other, our hearts racing. We looked at the telephone. I lifted the receiver and nervously said, *"Hello?"*

"Hi, I'm Joe Frank with Sunrise Memorial Services asking you to consider our prepaid funeral plans for those end-of-life decisions that we all must face at some point." The recording continued, but Jan was already puzzled by the growing smile on my face. After I shared with her "God's answer", we just couldn't stop laughing. Well, so much for solicited answers to prayer.

We made the decision to do the surgery in Dallas. Hannah stayed with Jan as Sara, Martha, Jonathan, and I drove back to Dallas on Sunday afternoon. My leg was still hurting. Earlier that day we had attended worship at First Baptist Church of Houston, where the pastor set aside a special moment of prayer for us. After the service, several deacons surrounded us in a private room and, laying their hands on us, prayed for healing, specifically mentioning my leg and Jan's lungs.

Back in Dallas, I left the kids in our new mission home while I drove my brother's car back to his house. I stayed a few minutes with him, my only sibling, telling him about the likelihood of my cancer having already spread to my leg and elsewhere. We had buried our mother just a few years back, and now this. It was a sad moment.

A couple from the church drove me back to the mission house in Dallas. It was then that I stared out the window at the nighttime, thinking about a comment Martha had made the previous day while we played in a Houston park. *"Dad, if heaven is such a wonderful place, why do people try so hard, with medicines and stuff, to stay here?"*

Yeah, why do we try so hard?

It was difficult for Jan not to be there for me and for the kids during my surgery. In her May 18 prayer letter, she wrote:

> Please keep praying for my healing and for Mark's as he faces his kidney surgery tomorrow. I have been discouraged by my slow healing. The Lord knows how anxious I am to be well so I can be in Dallas when Mark is dismissed from the Hospital. I have had many fears on how we will manage all this when I'm not healed

myself and can't really take care of Mark. But Psalm 34 makes me take heart. *"The righteous will never lack for any good thing"* The same scripture also reminds me that He will rescue me from all my fears. *"The righteous man may have many troubles but the Lord delivers him from them all."*

That same Tuesday morning in Dallas, I was alone in the house. Friends had picked up the kids the previous day, offering to keep them for as long as needed. I recall waking up and walking to the kitchen. My leg wasn't hurting! I thumped it, turned it, and jumped on it. No pain! Hmmm, I remembered the deacons in Houston.

On Wednesday morning, another friend from the church drove me to the hospital. I was so grateful my surgeon was a Christian. He prayed for me and for the surgery before they rolled me into the surgical area.

The surgery lasted a couple of hours. My first post surgical awareness was when they removed my catheter. An odd sensation.

I also remember my brief stay in the recovery room. Across from me, in another bed, a teenager's leg hung in a brace. The boy was large, but no where near as big as his 300+ pound mother who sat beside him in a stuffed chair. For breakfast, she ate a large bag of corn chips and drank a coke (not even a diet one). Lunch was the same, except she substituted the corn chips with potato chips.

"Here I was," I thought, *"with lines and tubes hanging out from me like a spider web, trapped among all these machines. I avoid junk food. I eat nutritiously. I've watched my weight carefully, and I am the one here with cancer. Lord,"* I said with a wry smile that only He could see, *"life just isn't fair."*

The surgeon visited me in the hospital the next morning. As I slowly sat up in bed, he gave me the good news and the bad news. The good news was that the kidney tumor, though large, was self-contained. He was able to routinely remove the tumor and the kidney without any complication. The bad news was that the two lymph nodes he had removed both tested positive for cancer cells. This was enough to officially stage my cancer at IV, the final stage. Well, at least we had a little life insurance.

Jan and I had learned long ago to look for God's *fingerprints* on our lives, especially during times of adversity. One of the biggest needs for missionaries returning to the States, other than housing, is a car. A godly lady from First Baptist Church of Houston, upon hearing our story, gave her car for us to use while we were in the States.

David finished his final exams for that semester and flew to Houston. Jan's drainage tubes were taken out and she was finally released for travel. David got the car, then drove Jan and Hannah to Dallas. Our friends brought back Sara, Martha, and Jonathan. The next day, I was released from the hospital. We were all together again.

An Eventful Summer

Even before my stitches were removed, Jan and I hit the research books. Jan was intelligent; I was curious. We wanted to know what caused our cancers and how were we going to treat them. We read books, searched the web, and talked to lots of folks. We learned that cancer was mostly the result of increased toxins in our environment and a decrease of essential nutrients in our foods. We learned that melanoma cancer and kidney cancer were biological siblings, their tumors sharing many immunological similarities.

One fact about our cancers became painfully clear. Traditional radiation and chemotherapy didn't usually work for either one.   The most common form of treatment for melanoma and kidney cancer was surgery and observation. Watch and wait, and hope the cancer doesn't grow back. But we were not content with doing nothing. The research continued.

It didn't take us long to search outside of traditional, allopathic medicine, and into the realm of alternative, or naturopathic medicine. We waded in carefully, cautiously, knowing that there were a lot of unregulated practitioners out there who were perhaps more shrewd with money than with medicine. We had the advantage of not being desperate. If the

Lord was ready to take us home to be with Him, we were ready. But we felt responsible for these temples of the Holy Spirit. So we prayed; we read.

Based on our research and on the knowledge of trusted friends, we chose a daily regiment of glyco- and phyto-nutrients, along with fish oil and enzymes. It was explained to us that many of these nutrients were just no longer in our western diets. After tasting some of these powdered concoctions, I knew why they were no longer in our diet! But I took my medicine anyway like a good boy.

Jan began making weekly trips to a nearby doctor for an immune system booster I.V. drip. Jan also agreed to do an FDA approved immunotherapy treatment of daily interferon I.V. infusions. Studies showed that this treatment didn't prolong life, but merely delayed the cancer's reoccurrence.

Jan's prayer letters during this time often read more like a Christian medical manual:

> I would ask prayer that the side effects not be so debilitating; particularly pray protection over my bone marrrow (damage here affects the white blood cells, red blood cells and platelets; I have had problems with anemia this past year) and liver (as the body's main detoxifying organ, it gets hit pretty hard). I have different elements of my battle plan to help me keep my body detoxed, but it depends on me having the energy to do them. I am claiming Psalm 41:3 *"The Lord nurses them when they are sick and eases their pain and discomfort.*

For the whole month of July, I took Jan on daily trips to the hospital for one hour infusion treatments. Jan experienced minimal side effects, other than sleeping through most of the day, as well as through the night. Always the missionary, Jan asked for prayer in her letters that, *"the light and love of Jesus will radiate from my infusion room."*

Another matter that concerned us was the view some of our Filipino friends and co-workers had toward suffering. They, like many in the U.S., would sometimes view sickness and disease the same way as the "friends" of the Old Testament sufferer, Job. *"God must be against you." "You must have done something to anger Him." "Sickness is surely God's punishment; a divine curse."*

Though we had tried to teach a Biblical view of suffering, it was time for a reminder. I spent the day of June 12, digging through the notes of my May 2 sermon, and wrote a long letter which I titled *God and Cancer.* In it, I gave some Biblical reasons why our cancers may have occurred. (see Appendix 1)

In one of her letters, Jan wrote, *"I have never wondered why this happened, but have asked God what does He want us to learn from it, and as I have shared before, I want Him to be glorified through it all. God isn't finished with us yet! We are telling people the good news that no matter what happens, we have a mighty God who walks with us every step of the way. And that is a joy that is indescribable."*

In mid July, we received a telephone call from Steve Blow, columnist for the Dallas Morning News. He had heard our story and wanted to do a write up about us. A photographer came by the house; she was from the Philippines. We enjoyed sharing with her as she snapped about a hundred pictures of us in casual poses. Of course only one picture would go with the story.

Steve Blow visited us a few days later and spent about an hour interviewing us as the girls worked in the kitchen, within hearing distance. We were glad to share our testimony, humbled by the attention, and appreciative of what he wrote. The article came out in early August. (see Appendix 2)

Jan and I were realistic enough to know that our time with the children might be short. One big issue we didn't have to worry about was who would be our children's legal guardians if we both were gone. Soon after David was born, and before we first left for the Philippines, Jan and I had considered the possibilities of what could happen to us on the mission field. We approached our very dear friends, Doug and Selah Helms, and asked if they would be our children's adopted parents, if anything happened to both of us.

They agreed. Over the years, our families have stayed in close contact. In fact, their oldest son was now David's roommate in college. Of course, Jan and I wanted very much to continue our role as parents. We love our children. But if we couldn't, we had complete confidence in Doug and Selah, knowing their values mirrored ours. Having this agreement gave Jan and I freedom to trust God with whatever He wanted to do in our lives.

Since our time might be limited, Jan and I wanted to do two things that summer. One was to get a nice, updated family picture. (The picture you see on the back cover was the result of that wish.) Secondly, we wanted to take a family vacation to Yellowstone National Park. This had been a dream of ours for years, and now was the time to do it.

By the first of August, Jan had finished her one month of high-dose interferon treatments. She was ready for a break from the immunotherapy regimen of daily infusions that left her tired and sleepy. So on August 9, we loaded up the car and headed to Wyoming, leaving behind prayer requests that our cancers wouldn't interfere in any way with our family vacation.

Jan's father and stepmother joined us for the trip. We spent four beautiful days in Grand Teton National Park, some of us hiking, others canoeing or sightseeing. Another four days were spent in Yellowstone, all of us enjoying the scenic overlooks and the short interpretive walks. Twice on the last day we stopped for a family of bears as they passed in front of our car. It was a wonderful vacation.

We arrived back in Fort Worth on the 20th, feeling tired but relatively good. We celebrated David's birthday on the 22nd, then he headed back to college to begin his second semester. I was scheduled for more scans on the 23rd, anxious to see the results, especially concerning my left leg.

Waiting

The fall brought with it some good health news. My scans were clear of any cancer. The spot on my leg had not grown; the pain never returned.   On September 22, my orthopedic oncologist (bone cancer specialist), concluded that the "suspicious focal point" was of some unknown benign origin and for me not to worry about it.

The questionable spots in Jan's lungs were not growing either. After her October 7 scan it was concluded that these were not cancerous, but probably some benign souvenir bacterial growth leftover from our time in the tropics. Harmless. Her scans were also showing no evidence of any cancer elsewhere. We were obviously pleased.

A little biology lesson here. It is usually incorrect to say that a recent cancer victim is disease free. Instead, the better term is NED (No Evidence of Disease).   Often, after cancer surgery to remove a tumor, tiny cancer cells can travel through the blood stream or lymph system to other areas of the body and start new tumors. It may take months or years before they grow large enough to be detected by imaging machines like the CT (computerized tomography) scanner, or an MRI (magnetic resonance imaging).

Cancers vary in their rate of tumor growth. Breast cancer tumors may take several years before they are large enough to be seen by a scanner. More aggressive cancers, like ours, will usually show new tumor growth within two to three years. But every cancer patient always hopes that their surgery, radiation, or chemotherapy treatment killed ALL the cancer cells.

It is also helpful to know that when a cancer metastasizes (spreads beyond the original site), it carries with it the same characteristics of the original cancer. So if my leg bone had been cancerous, it would have still been called kidney cancer, but in my leg bone. If the spots in Jan's lungs had been metastasized melanoma, it would still have been called skin cancer, but in her lungs.

Jan and I knew that, even though our scans were not detecting any cancerous growth, we were still at high risk for reoccurrence, meaning we likely had cancer cells that were starting new tumors, but were still too small to be seen by scanners. However, we didn't want to be inactive, twiddling our thumbs waiting to see if our cancers would return. All summer long and into the fall, we were in frequent contact with our mission board, pleading with them for permission to return to the Philippines.

In the meantime, though, life had to continue for our family. Because of the many uncertainties we were facing, this committed, die-hard home schooling mom and dad made the reluctant choice of enrolling Jonathan and Martha in a nearby public elementary school. We had heard so many negative stories about public schools that, until now, we never thought of it as an option.

But again, God knew what we needed and where we needed to be. Jan and I made appointments in August to meet the principal and teachers of the nearby school. To our surprise, most of them were active Christians! Knowing that we were living nearby, they had even posted the Dallas Morning News article on their school bulletin board.

Martha and Jonathan had a very positive experience in the school. Their teachers affirmed both of them over and over for their strength of character and their strong academic abilities. Both easily made the honor roll.

Sara and Hannah continued their schooling at home, both doing well with their grades and tests. Hannah took cake decorating classes and worked some at the church library. Both girls were a huge help with meals and house cleaning chores.

Jan and I stayed occupied with medical matters, including frequent doctor visits. Jan was developing quite a rapport with her doctors. As a biology major, she could talk intelligently and thoroughly with them. Having a gregarious personality, she was also rather entertaining.

"During one visit," Jan recalled, *"my oncologist walked in the room. "Good afternoon, Mrs. Moses. You're looking so good!" (One of the fun things about this cancer business is that when I see people, they always exclaim on how good I look. More compliments than I've had in a lifetime!) I responded to him, "Well, as Eliza Doolittle in My Fair Lady said, "I warsted my face and hands before I cum, I did."*

By this time, Jan had chosen not to restart the interferon infusions. Their limited benefits just didn't justify the physical and financial costs. Jan didn't want to sleep through the fall while the world passed by. Aided by generous gifts from dear friends, we did continue our neutricuitical regimen.

We enjoyed immensely the fellowship of First Baptist of Dallas. They loved on us till our hearts were ready to burst with gratitude. Jan concluded her October 8, 2004, prayer letter with this:

> And God is so faithful to send a "glory drop" our way whenever my emotions start to drag. We received prayer quilts this week from Calvary Baptist in Brenham, Texas as a visual reminder of their prayers. I am going to take mine with me to church this Sunday night as the choir at FBC Dallas sings, *Somebody's Praying Me Through*. I figure I'll just cry the entire service, so I'm taking a box of tissues with me. This is where we are -- we know that day-by-day, month by month, we have peace, security, joy -- because so many are praying us through this adventure. Thank you so much for your part in our physical healing and our emotional and spiritual health. To God Be the Glory!

Returning to the Philippines

The moment we left the Philippines, it was our heart's desire to return. One, we never sensed an end to our call as missionaries. Second, Southern Baptists were still paying us a salary and we felt guilty that we weren't doing our job. Third, we missed our Filipino friends. As Hannah said in a letter, *"They are the true heroes in the ministry as they work with so little physical compensation and under so many hardships."*

Fourth, the Philippines was our home, where all our children had grown up, where our friends, dogs, and memories still lived. Finally, we wanted to return because the temperature was starting to get cold and we missed sunning at the beach while folks here shivered in the winter. Aren't we awful!

On a late October day, cheers and shouts of joy erupted from our home after we received final clearance from our mission board to return to the Philippines. Packing began immediately. We gave notice to Jonathan and Martha's teachers that they would leave soon and not finish the semester. Both of their classes had a sweet goodbye party just for them.

It was decided that I would go first with Sara and Jonathan, so that I could prepare the house and attend our Associational Meeting. Hannah and Martha would come with Jan after they celebrated Thanksgiving with her dad in Virginia. Can you sense our excitement in Jan's November 6 prayer letter?

> We are awed, that only 6 months after both of us were diagnosed with stage 3 / possible stage 4 cancers, that the IMB medical department has given Mark and I clearance to return to the Philippines. WOW!!! Isn't God amazing? This could only be a work of His grace and power and your prayerful support and encouragement. We had been praying that He would guide the medical department and our regional leadership and we trust that this is His will for us at this time.
>
> Now don't stop praying for us! We realize that both of us are at high risk for reoccurrence because we both had lymph node involvement but our future is in His hands. We feel that He is not finished with us yet in the Philippines. Pray for our physical, spiritual, and emotional protection as you have prayed for our health.
>
> We will return to our home in Iloilo City where a friend has been staying in the home and taking care of the dogs for us. We will be following up with oncologists in Manila (capital of the Philippines) every 3 months. It is a 1 hour plane ride (or an 18 hour boat trip!). I will also see a dermatologist there. If we need to have scans done, there is a brand new CT scan machine that was donated to the Baptist hospital in our city of Iloilo. (Even with the plane ride, medical costs in the Philippines are much less than in the U.S. so we feel that we are being good stewards of the Lord's money). We will continue taking our immune boosting supplements as well as watching our diet and exercise.
>
> Please pray that God would give us wisdom on any environmental toxins that could have contributed to our cancers. We have some ideas as to possible causes, but don't know where to go for testing or how to fix any

problems. But God knows and has faithfully given us direction on things like this in the past.

Thank you for your faithful prayers for the children. They have been secure and even joyful through this whole experience. They have seen God's blessings through His people and experienced His love and provision. We praise God that David will be able to join us in the Philippines at Christmas due to the generosity of some friends in Georgia who bought his ticket.

While this has not been a normal furlough (now called stateside assignment) because we have not been able to travel and speak in churches (which we really enjoy doing!), there have been new experiences that have brought us joy. One of them has been to worship at FBC of Dallas. Music, choirs, and orchestra are always such a blessing to us on furloughs and it has been an exciting experience at FBC.

Another blessing during furloughs is listening to God's word, and again we have been encouraged and challenged by Dr. Brunson's messages. Because we have been at FBC, we have "expanded our territory" of dear friends that we have met at FBC and feel that it was God's plan to have brought us here for this unique time. This FBC mission home was so convenient for a 1-car family with lots of travel to doctor appointments.

We will "divide and conquer" for our return. Mark, along with Sara and Jonathan will arrive in the Philippines on Monday November 15. Jan, along with Hannah and Martha, will clean up, finish Hannah's cake decorating class and visit with Jan's family in Virginia before leaving on December 1.

Now, we hope that from now on, we can focus once again on the people group that God has called us to serve. We don't know what He has been doing in the lives of the church members, pastors, and church leaders in our area.

Pray that they would be challenged to live each day as if it were their last. Pray that we would all have an urgency and boldness in our witness. Pray that, even now, the Holy Spirit is preparing the hearts of those that we need to speak with and that He will lead us to them.

"I (we) *waited patiently for the LORD: He turned to*

me (us) and heard my (our) cry.   He lifted me out of the slimy pit... He set my feet on a rock... Many will see and fear and put their trust in the LORD... Many, O LORD my God, are the wonders you have done. The things you planned for us no one can recount to you; were I to speak and tell of them, they would be too many to declare.... I speak of your faithfulness and salvation. I do not conceal your love and your truth from the great assembly... May all who seek you rejoice and be glad in you; may those who love your salvation always say, "The LORD be exalted!" (Psalm 40)

Indeed, may the LORD be exalted!   As you worship tomorrow, praise Him for His faithfulness and salvation!

Four days later, our continued excitement elicited another letter from Jan:

Oh Victory in Jesus! My Savior, forever. He sought me and bought me, with His redeeming love.   He loved me ere I knew Him and all my love is due Him...

What a joy to attend worship and sing praises openly to God. Greater yet is the awareness that God chose us to be His children -- He took the initiative to reach out to us. This always boggles my mind.

If ever Mark and I ask ourselves, "Why me?", it is in reflection on this truth. "Why me, Lord? Why have you made yourself known to me? Why did you choose me to be your ambassador in the Philippines? We are so unworthy to be your servants."

We are continually aware of the privilege it is to be His missionaries. And we are very thankful and grateful to Southern Baptists for their support through the Lottie Moon Christmas Offering. We regret that we have not been able to visit in churches and share that message with you. We are also grateful for the Cooperative Program (a portion of your weekly tithes goes to CP which funds up to 50% of International Mission Board budget). These two offerings are the lifeline of our financial support and we wish we could tell you that in person.

I always want to share with churches how very essential your prayer support is. We have known that in the past, shared that on previous furloughs and in e-mails, but we cannot emphasize it enough. We have literally these past 7 months been strengthened and upheld by your prayers. I tell people that in tough times, one thing that keeps us going is knowing that we are not alone, but that the great family of God -- many of whom we have never met face to face -- comes boldly into the throne of God to intercede on our behalf.

"In our hearts, we felt the sentence of death. But this happened that we might not rely on ourselves but on God, who raises the dead. He has delivered us from such a deadly peril, and He will deliver us. On Him we have set our hope that He will continue to deliver us, as you help us by your prayers. Then many will give thanks on our behalf for the gracious favor granted us in answer to the prayers of many" (2 Corinthians 1: 9-11).

This says it all! God is good and He is Sovereign.

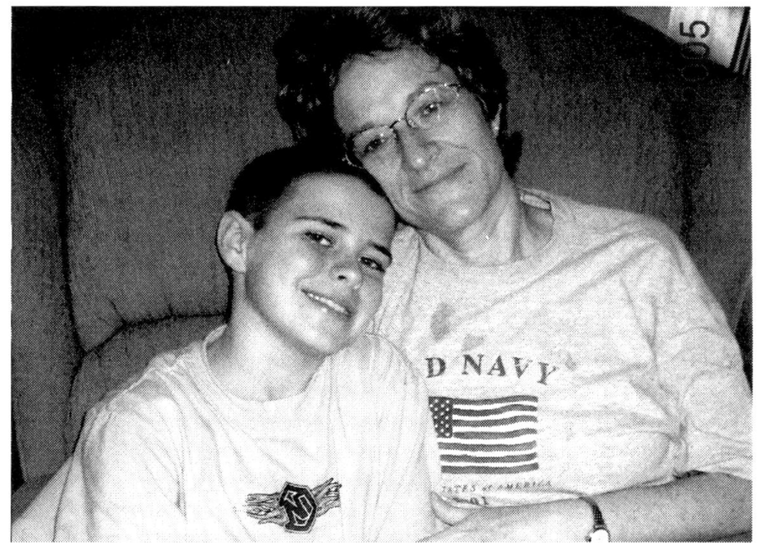

Jonathan with Mom

Chapter 4: THE CANCER RETURNS

It is always a mixed bag of emotions that we carry off the plane upon arriving in the Philippines. Manila is crowded, noisy, and polluted. The heat and humidity feels like an opened oven. There are beggars on the sidewalks, traffic clogging the streets, and sewage filling the rivers. Not the place for pleasant memories.

Another plane ride will take us to Iloilo City. A bit cleaner, but still noisy and crowded. There will be the daily challenge of trying to stay cool in the tropical heat, and the inconvenience of dealing with frequent brown-outs (loss of electricity). Food from the market will have to be carefully washed. Our open-air home will require frequent cleaning. The ministry needs of three church associations will be waiting at my doorstep.

So why were we so excited to come? Ah, because this is where the Lord is at work, on the frontiers of His kingdom, winning the lost and maturing the saved. This is where we have seen God change lives, where the Holy Spirit has delivered men and women trapped in superstitious fears and transformed them into shining trophies of His grace. This is where our family has grown up and grown close, away from the distracting, worldly influences of American culture. This is where God has called us, to a land not our own, but wholly His.

Getting Settled

By early December, 2004, we were all together again in our home in Iloilo. There were church problems to deal with, schooling to start up, and Christmas to prepare for. Jan and I had a new appreciation for time, knowing cancer could return at any moment for one or both of us. We had prepared an action plan involving various scenarios in case one of us had a reoccurrence. It was a plan we hoped never to use, but we were realistic enough to know we probably would.

In a December 7 letter to a friend, Jan explained our situation:

Well, I am home now and reality hits. You can imagine a house that has been open to dust, humidity, mice, and bugs for 7 months. We had a couple staying here who took care of basics, but not walls, windows and closets so we have quite a clean-up job to do. Ants are living in my closet and clothes, cockroaches have taken over the bottom cabinets, Hannah has already found that many of her clothes have mildewed. Thankfully we are having "cool" weather (upper 70s / lower 80s), so it is tolerable to work but we need some bright sunshine if we are going to wash and dry everything before putting it up (we have never had a dryer).

I need you to pray as I go room by room, closet by closet, box by box. It is not as if we just pick up our lives where we left off, plan for our next furlough in X years, order curriculum for the next school year, etc. We don't know what tomorrow -- or the next set of scans will bring. We are not fearful, yet we need to be prepared.

Mark said it was overwhelming to him last May when he was trying to get some basics sorted in case we didn't come back. He wants me to downsize as much as possible. Yet I have a tendency to hang on to stuff -- no Wal-mart to run to if you need it!

But I see his point. The mission board has graciously allowed us to return, which we have asked people to pray for the Lord to give them wisdom. The missionaries here on the field were VERY surprised that they let us return with our high possibility of reoccurrence. We need to be prepared to return to the U.S. at any time.

Thankfully, the Lord KNOWS and without giving us the details, He can direct me item by item, box by box on what to keep and what to give away. These decisions tax the mind and sap the energy! I still feel a tendency to hold on to things, because if we have to return to the U.S. due to the cancer, then we will have no job or insurance or money to buy stuff. Then I remind myself of God's promise that I claimed this past June when things looked very bleak for both of us -- that I've never seen the righteous forsaken OR THEIR CHILDREN BEGGING FOR BREAD.

And indeed God's people showered us with blessings and we lacked nothing (did I tell you that we never had to buy toilet paper or paper towels from June until we left because we were given so much!). And I remind myself of all that He provided in allowing us to live in that lovely mission house and for the kids to have friends and great teachers at the elementary school. Truly He can do far more than we can even think or imagine! (I think I better write that verse in big letters to hover over me while I sort and pack).

I will be asking people to pray in bits and pieces since I can't send out a group email. In transporting our old computer (poor thing doesn't handle flights well), once again it crashed and we lost everything -- including our prayer email address list. Fortunately, I have a printed copy of our address book, but the thought of typing 600 addresses isn't high on my list of things to do right now!...

Jan stayed busy on the home front as I involved myself in ministry activities. The Lord was opening up new areas for church planting. Several of our older churches were catching the vision of multiplying themselves into new churches. We were seeing many of our church leaders maturing in their relationship with the Lord. One evidence for this was hearing some of our leaders speak about becoming missionaries themselves. As Jan explained:

> After a visit to Thailand in 1999, I was challenged anew by the lostness in so many of the countries in Asia. Our Pacific Rim region extends from the north in Japan and Korea through the Southeast Asia countries of Thailand and surrounding countries down to Indonesia and Papua New Guinea -- about 17% of the world's unreached population.
>
> But in South Asia -- the countries of India, Pakistan, Nepal, Bhutan, Bangladesh, Sri Lanka -- contain almost 35% of the world's unreached population. Even if you read mission magazines and pray regularly for these countries, you cannot really imagine the lostness until you have physically been there. What a contrast to the hope, love, and security that we have in Jesus Christ.
>
> When we went on furlough (stateside assignment) in 2000, I asked myself if we should leave our "comfort" zone of the Philippines and go to one of these countries.
>
> But the direction that I felt God leading, and what I shared with churches that furlough, that my role here in the Philippines would be to encourage and help Filipinos to go to these countries. They have so many skills in language, adaptability, and lifestyle to help them. And God has placed Filipinos throughout the world as "tentmakers", earning their own living (8 million Filipinos work overseas).
>
> Our Mindanao Visayas Convention has sent out three Filipino missionaries this year. Filipinos are seeing God provide in amazing ways. We want to see workers go out as intentional missionaries -- tentmaking to earn their living, but going into these countries with a heart and vision to win the lost.

Indeed, we were seeing fruitfulness on various ministry fronts, from evangelistic responses to new church starts, from discipleship training to restored relationships. Jan and I were glad we had made the choice to return. But we constantly had our health concerns hanging over us.

In February, Jan and I joined hands together as we walked into Iloilo Mission Hospital for our regular check up and CT scans. Often we would joke with receptionists, suggesting they should give us a couple's discount. Two scans for the price of one, or, do one scan and get the next one free. But we never had any takers.

Our scans showed that we were still NED (no evidence of disease). We thanked the Lord and pressed on with our work. Jan woke one morning in mid March with a bit of nausea. But she dismissed it, as we had so often, as just another consequence of living in a third world, tropical country.

Work and Play

By March 19, we had reconstructed our address list and Jan was finally able to send out a newsletter:

The ole gray mare, she ain't what she used to be, ain't what she used to be.... many long years ago...

Well, that seems to be my theme song these days (and yes, my hair is gray!). Unpacking, organizing the house, homeschool, 3 trips to Manila, getting our email address list back up, etc. have taken my time and all seem to take me longer. Jonathan is impatient for things to "get back to normal". We have talked about the "bend" in our road and that life will never be exactly what it was "BC" -- before cancer...

People often ask how are Mark and I doing. We rejoice that our last check-ups were both clear with **no evidence of cancer**. We are following up with oncologists here in Iloilo. Mark is feeling great and I am feeling better as we continue to adjust my thyroid medication. Our next set of CT scans is at the end of May. The Baptist hospital here in our city had a brand new CT scan machine donated last year that produces excellent pictures (wasn't God good to prepare that for us?).

Several people in the U.S. expressed a concern that we should stay in the U.S. where we could monitor our diet better and perhaps have better follow-up, less exposure to toxins, etc. I don't know about that, but I do know that all of this is NOT just about us. While we will do what we can where God has called us, our goal in life is not to keep the Moseses alive, but to glorify God and be His ministers of reconciliation. We have a message of hope to share with so many who have no hope! Sometimes I get tired of writing about us but yet I know we need your prayers as this is a spiritual battle and that you care about us. So thank you for your patience as we get through this and onto the bigger picture that God sees.

As you can tell, it has been a year of change -- some major, some minor. But life is like that, isn't it? It's another theme that I keep coming back to in my bedtime talks with Jonathan. There is always change and I don't think most people like change, to be shaken out of their comfort zone. But in the midst of changes, there is a constant -- God. His character, His love, His mercy, His faithfulness -- it is always there.

Psalm 46 talks of changes -- physical changes in the earth (tsunamis?), changes in governments and nations, changes in peace and order. But the psalmist starts with an absolute unchanging unshakeable truth -- *"God is our refuge and strength, an ever-present help in trouble. Therefore we will not fear even though..."* (You can fill in the blank with whatever changes you are going through).

And the psalmist ends with *"Be still and know that I am God; I will be exalted among the nations."* We can rest secure in God and that is where we are.

Easter was a pleasant celebration. Jan fixed her traditional meal of turkey, dressing, mashed potatoes, seven-layered salad, and pumpkin pie. We chatted with David on the telephone. The nausea Jan had felt in mid March was still bothering her. But there were several possibilities as to what could be causing it. Besides, her February scan had been clear.

April did not offer us time for rest. We had two huge events to prepare for and participate in. One was our semi annual Association Meeting. I was the main speaker and would be introducing our new discipleship training materials designed to guide us in implementing CPM (Church Planting Movements), a recent worldwide strategy emphasis of the International Mission Board.

Second, the Triennial Assembly of the Philippine Women's Missionary Union was to be held in Iloilo. Once every three years, our Philippine WMU holds a nationwide convention. Our city was the host for this convention. A rare honor, it also meant a lot of work for our ladies, including Jan.

Despite all the work (and her persistent nausea), Jan still found time for a little pleasure. It had been one year since the beginning of our cancer adventure, so Hannah suggested we should celebrate. We had a family friend whose husband owned one of the nicest hotels in Iloilo. She made an offer to us of a free night in the family suite, complete with a complimentary massage and a free breakfast. And, the room had a Jacuzzi.

Now, we missionary folk live a simple lifestyle. We ain't accustomed to the nicer things in life. We knew what a Jacuzzi was, but had never seen one, much less used one. Now was our chance for some cultural comfort. With her bathing suit on, Jan filled the tub and poured in some Bubble Bath, a lot of Bubble Bath. After all, it was a big tub.

The kids were outside the bathroom, waiting their turn. They heard the click of a switch, the roar of the air jets, the gurgling of the water, and then Mom screamed. But the scream was quickly followed by hilarious laughter as the suds started seeping out from under the door. Jan was having a grand time in a bathroom filled with Bubble Bath. Soon, all the kids were in the bathroom, dancing and sliding on the floor as Mom soaked in a sea of bubbles.

Not Feeling Well

A few days before the Bubble Bath celebration, Jan had written her doctor in the States:

> I have had nausea the last 3 weeks and some fatigue. (Changed thyroid medications in February and for about 2 weeks felt my old energy coming back but that didn't last long! TSH elevated again.) The nausea is all day, no appetite, and doesn't seem to be related to anything that I eat. But if I do eat, then I feel better for about 30 - 45 minutes before the nausea returns. I am not vomiting, just an ongoing queasy stomach. I have never experienced anything like this before.

A blood test showed her LDH blood levels were elevated. Jan suspected problems with her liver, and possibly a reoccurrence of cancer. But an ultrasound on April 15 did not detect anything abnormal.

Still the nausea continued and Jan grew weaker. On April 29, she wrote again to a doctor:

> My fatigue seems to be getting better, which may just be time as my U.S. doctor suggested. Or maybe I am just getting used to operating at a lower energy level!
>
> On March 15, I suddenly had nausea. It has been constant since then and I have no appetite and a bad taste always in my mouth. When I do eat, it seems that my food and vitamins just sit in my stomach like a lead balloon. I have lost 7 pounds in the last 2 weeks. I retch every time that I drink my medication powder.
>
> I had an endoscopy done this week and there is some inflammation in the stomach, so the doctor is calling it mild gastritis and has prescribed proton pump inhibitor drug and antinausea. I don't like the side effects or toxicity on the liver (one of my liver enzymes is elevated -- over twice the upper limit of normal) and so haven't started them yet.

About this time we had a visit from a trained therapist, sent by the Mission Board to evaluate our situation. They wanted to know how we were coping with the stress of knowing our cancers might return at anytime. They also wanted to know how the children were adjusting to the real possibility of their parents dying from cancer. The visit went fine and he concluded that all of us were coping amazingly well.

Jan made some observations in her notebook:

The therapist had the viewpoint that tragedy was "bad" and therefore had to be "worked through." But from a Biblical viewpoint, we are to count adversity as *"pure joy"* (James 1). *"The righteous will have many problems, but the Lord delivers them."* The therapist wondered if our children had regressed because of our situation. He didn't consider the possibility that maybe they had grown in maturity because of it. He said we needed to "settle in" where we can get proper help when we need it; to go to our comfort zone. But after 19 years here in the Philippines, this is our comfort zone and home for the children.

One of the last projects I had with David before he left for college in 2004 was to write a research paper on the topic of *suffering*. My goal was to give him a biblical foundation in understanding God's purposes for his trials BEFORE they came. He learned that our first response to trials is not to run away from them, but to allow God to accomplish His purposes through them. And His purposes almost always involved maturing us in some aspect of our character. He learned that we could either let trials defeat us, or they could be marvelous opportunities for spiritual growth. Perhaps it was training like this that helped our children adjust so well to our cancer adventure.

Jan knew that her continued nausea and elevated blood levels could be caused by a reoccurrence of cancer. But we were counting on her clear ultrasound as evidence that it wasn't cancer. On May 8, Jan wrote:

Thanks for the prayers last week. I had the endoscopy without sedation -- the doctor numbed my throat and then told me when to swallow. Not too much different than the nausea I've been having and I just practiced the deep breathing / relaxation that helped with 5 childbirths.

The endoscopy just showed mild stomach inflammation (gastritis); the doctor doesn't know if this is causing the nausea / weight loss but she prescribed drugs. However these anti-nausea and anti-ulcer medicines both have effects on the liver, so I haven't started them yet. I have really made myself eat a little something every few hours this past week and so the weight loss has stopped (although everyone has been commenting on how nice I look!).

One of my liver enzymes (LDH -- a nonspecific marker but can be elevated in melanoma) is now 3 times the upper limit of normal, so I will probably have a CT scan this week.

The day after Jan's CT scan, while a friend had gone to the hospital to pick up the results, I sent out an email that marked a sort of milestone in our ministry:

I promised Jan I would write an e-mail when the training materials were done. Well, today they got done. The project began in December, 2001, when it was very apparent we needed simple, reproducible evangelistic and discipleship materials in the local Ilonggo dialect. It took a year to put the English version together, then nearly two and a half years to translate it. Of course, nearly a year of that was our health interruption last year.

Not only was the translation finished last week, but we were able to print them at a very low cost. It will take another two days to fold, sort, and wrap the materials, but they will be ready by the time we have our first CPM (Church Planting Movement) leadership training this Saturday. Well, I have learned that nothing ever goes as planed, but I would appreciate you praying with me that our church leaders will have a burden to reach the lost and disciple the saved.

I still do a good bit of traveling. Last Friday, I drove two and a half hours north to speak at a college Baccalaureate service, then traveled west for over three hours through mountain and coastal roads, plus an evening thunder storm, to counsel with a group of young people till 1 a.m. about a church problem they were facing. The storm had caused a black out so we ate and talked by candlelight, then slept in the tropical heat without the benefit of a fan. Early in the morning I began the five hour journey back to Iloilo. Ah, the joys of ministry.

Moments after the above email was sent out, our friend arrived back from the hospital with Jan's CT scan results. Sara, Hannah, and I were working in the schoolroom when Jan came in and read the report: *"The liver and spleen are enlarged with multiple various sized hypodense nodules..."* Mom's cancer had returned.

Being pro-active, Jan's first thoughts related to details, such as what reports will we need, which doctors should we consult, what therapies can we consider. After a few minutes of technical talk, there was a moment of silence. We looked at each other. The reality of the moment hit us; we knew what this meant. A tear here and there began to fall.

We would have to pack and leave, this time almost certain never to return. Metastatic melanoma spreads aggressively. It is almost never curable. Death usually comes in a matter of months.

The tears flowed.

Leaving Once Again

That evening we decided not to tell anyone else just yet. Tomorrow was Jonathan's birthday, and this was not a present we wanted to give him. Jan also didn't want to notify the Mission Board, knowing their first instructions would be to fly to the States immediately. Our annual mission meeting in June was to be in Thailand. Jan, always putting her family first, didn't want the kids to miss an opportunity to experience another culture. With the thoughts of having to uproot our family once again, Jan seriously considered spending her last days on earth in Iloilo. After all, this was our comfort zone; this was home.

But as the week wore on, her nausea worsened. Jan could actually see the bulge of her enlarging spleen. We realized that professional pain management would become an ever increasing want. We began saying goodbye to our dreams of visiting Thailand. As the pros and cons were weighed, the scales tipped more and more toward the side of us returning to Texas.

We shared the news with Martha and Jonathan. On May 18, we called David. Jan then called our mission board doctor and told him. The next day, Jan told everyone else:

We all celebrated when the translation and printing of Mark's discipleship materials were done last week. David asked, *"That was a big project. What is next on Dad's agenda?"* I told him that I was sure that God had something else for us to do.

That something else may not be in our plans nor our desires. I had a CT scan done and it showed that there are nodules in my liver and spleen. (The great news is that my liver enzymes are all in the normal range so the liver is still functioning well). The doctor here is assuming metastasized melanoma, but we have sent the scans to MD Anderson Cancer Center for a second opinion.

Lord willing, I will have a liver biopsy done in Manila on Monday May 23... We so appreciate your faithful prayers and concerns. We will just continue to rest in the Lord during this time of waiting to see what direction our lives will take. Please pray for all the doctors involved to have wisdom, for tests to be done accurately and in a timely manner, and for us, the IMB medical department and regional office to know God's direction.

"How excellent is Thy lovingkindness, O God! Therefore the children of men put their trust under the shadow of Thy wings" Psalm 36:7.

The following week, Jan flew with Sara to Manila and into the caring hands of our fellow missionaries there. Jan had the liver biopsy, initial readings confirming melanoma cancer. A bone scan revealed probable cancerous growth in both legs and arms. An ultrasound detected abnormalities in her kidneys.

While there, she began taking a prescribed oral chemotherapy drug that couldn't cure the cancer, but could possibly slow its progression.

Back in Iloilo, I was hurrying to finish several ministry projects while the kids began to pack. We knew by now that we would have to return to the States. Our mission board told us to pack with the assumption that we would not return.

When Jan flew back to Iloilo, she was obviously weakening. Still, her faith was focused on the Lord. On May 28, 2005, she wrote:

During my many tests in Manila this past week, I meditated on Psalm 139 and other Scriptures. When the interventional radiologist delicately guided the needle to the most accessible liver nodule, I reflected, *"O Lord, you have searched me and you know me. You know when I sit and when I rise... You discern my going out and my lying down; you are familiar with all my ways"* (Psalm 139: 2-3).

After the technician attached the electrodes to my brain for the EEG, I thought of how God knew already what was going on in there. *"You hem me in -- behind and before; you have laid your hand upon me. Such knowledge is too wonderful for me, too lofty for me to attain"* (vs. 5 - 6).

As the MRI machine banged and rattled my brain, I was comforted to remember, *"Where can I go from your spirit? Where can I flee from your presence? If I go up to the heavens, you are there; if I make my bed in the depths, you are there. If I rise on the wings of the dawn, if I settle on the far side of the sea, even there your hand will guide me, your right hand will hold me fast"* (vs. 7-10).

When the radiologist called me back for more bone scans of my arm, I thought, *"All the days ordained for me were written in your book before one of them came to be"* (vs. 16).

And what of the days ahead? It seems from the results that the cancer has returned with a vengeance. The liver biopsy was positive for melanoma. My liver has over 50% involvement, my spleen enlarged with large nodules. There are metastasis in the legs, hips and arms, especially the right arm at the original surgery site. We are shocked at the speed of it all (I had a normal ultrasound in April).

We are packing up this week to return to the U.S. How can you pray?

1. For Travel on June 4. I started chemotherapy Friday morning for 5 days in an effort to slow progression of the cancer. Hopefully, the side effects will not be too debilitating and I will be able to travel to Manila on June 3 for our early morning Northwest Airlines flight on the 4th. We have paid extra to get me a business class seat so that I can rest easier on the long (24 hour!) flight. Our thanks to FBC Dallas who sent us a love gift before we even knew that we would need it! Right now one of my ribs is very painful so pray that I can have a relatively pain-free flight. Particularly pray for the liver to continue functioning well (praise God it is still functioning amazingly well considering!).

2. Mark will stay here another week to finish packing and closing up things (and to have his next set of scans!!). As a recovering cancer patient himself, he felt it would be too stressful to try and get all of us out on the same day, so this gives him some additional time to pack and sell our belongings (and also frees me just to concentrate on getting on the airplane!).

3. For a house in Fort Worth. My oncologist has moved his clinic 30 minutes north of Dallas and the house that we lived in last year is not available. It seems that Dallas is closed to us at this time. So we want to be near family and friends in Ft. Worth. I am praying for a comfortable house in a safe and secure neighborhood where Jonathan can ride his bike and make friends. The Lord knows our needs but this is the first time I have had some desires also. I want a special place to have good family times.

4. We need a car. I know nothing about current prices,

styles, gasoline prices, and what is good for a family of 7. (Personally, my children had promised me a little bright yellow Volkswagen Beetle for when we retired...) Any advice, prayers, etc. appreciated.

5. An oncologist in Ft. Worth and God's leading on continued treatment.

6. Many decisions as we pack and sort from our 19 years of life in the Philippines. The International Mission Board is graciously paying for our crating and shipping. What a blessing -- takes some of the pressure off the "do we take this or not?" decisions.

7. For the children as they grieve the loss of their home and culture, friends, dogs, and parakeets. That we will have good closure on our years as a family here. It is hard to take time to "say good-bye" when we have so many immediate needs shouting to be done. For my father Bill Joness as he deals with seeing his daughter fight cancer (my mom died of breast cancer 17 years ago).

8. For constant electricity. This is our "summer" and it is hot. We have been having brown-outs for several hours every day. I get more nauseated in the heat. I am planning to hide out in our bedroom where we have an airconditioner -- as long as there is electricity! The heat, decisions, etc. make patience run out easier!

We praise God that there is no brain metastasis. We are so thankful that David arrived from the States this past Thursday and is helping with moving boxes and entertaining Jonathan. We are still trying to get him on the same flight as we are on (so he can be responsible for Jonathan and avoid a "Home Alone" situation while I am up in business class!).

Tomorrow, Jonathan and Martha will be baptized at the beach, as were their older siblings. We had been talking about it for some time. Pray that it is a special time for us all. It will be our "farewell party" with our church members. We had several pastors come by today to offer their support and prayers; we encouraged them to press on in the work of the Lord!

Your prayers, support, and love mean so very much. These past few weeks, many have shared how God has prompted them to pray for us. Thank you for responding to the Lord and being faithful to lift us up.

"How precious to me are your thoughts, O God! How vast is the sum of them! Were I to count them, they would outnumber the grains of sand. When I awake, I am still with you." (vs. 17 - 18). Resting in His mercy, Jan.

Always the Encourager

Palm trees covered the bamboo and thatched roof pavilion on the beach where our church family gathered on Sunday, June 2. A warm southern wind was whipping up waves as I led Martha and Jonathan into the waters of baptism. Jan savored it all. Later, testimonies were given, stories shared, and goodbye hugs were exchanged.

Strangely, leaving this time was not quite as traumatic as the year before. We had known that this day would likely come. We had emotionally envisioned it, mentally prepared for it. Still the goodbyes were hard.

A steady stream of visitors graced our house during the rest of the week as we sorted through our belongings, deciding what to pack, what to sell, and what to give away. Jan's nausea and fatigue limited her activity, but they wouldn't keep her down.

A missionary friend had introduced us to www.caring-bridge.org, a web site for families in crisis to share updates with friends. In our first entry on June 2, 2005, Jan shared:

We consider ourselves immensely privileged to have raised our family over here. Some say - you have given yourself to the Lord in his service in a far away land, and this is what you get? This is not our feeling; living here has not been a trial but a blessing! Raising our kids here has taught all of us the value of simplicity, how privileged and wealthy Americans are, and the practice of hospitality.

Our lives have been so enriched by living in another culture, maybe not enriched like most Americans are with church functions, soccer, and other programs, but enriched with values that we would never have learned in the States. My kids have grown up to have a bigger picture than just our lives, and have become aware about how the rest of the world lives. We are so grateful for the years God has abundantly blessed us with in the Philippines.

That night, Jan and I lay in bed, staring at the ceiling. The next day she and the kids were to leave Iloilo and then fly to the States. My back was aching terribly because of a sprain I had earned from lifting boxes. But Jan was hurting much, much more. By now her enlarged spleen was pressing against her lungs, hindering her breathing. She had begun vomiting. This responsible mother, who had worked all week sorting and packing in the tropical heat, was exhausted.

We talked for a few moments about what lay ahead. We spoke about funeral arrangements, her Memorial Service, and where she was to be buried. In the days ahead, her upbeat faith would lead some to think Jan was in denial about her condition. If they could only hear her speak now.

Soon, Jan drifted off to sleep. I continued to lay on my side, looking at this faithful lady I was so proud to call my wife. Earlier that day, a group of pastors and church leaders had come to encourage Jan and say goodbye. But instead, Jan was the one who encouraged them! *"Don't be sad for me,"* she told them, *"I know where I'm going. I am ready. God is not surprised by any of this. He knew before I was ever born that this day would come for me. I don't know what God is going to do, but I know I can trust Him with whatever lies ahead. And just as I can trust Him with this, I know you can trust Him with whatever struggles you face."*

I turned over my tear dampened pillow, closed my eyes, and talked to God.

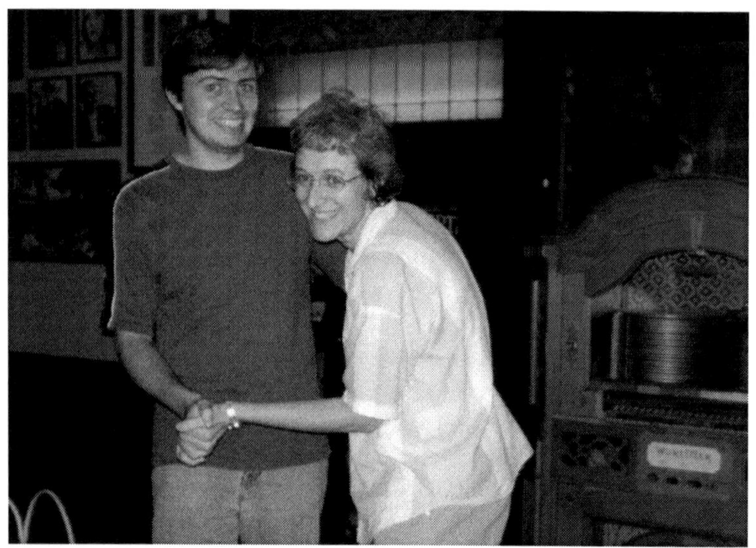

Doing a jig with David at the dude ranch

Chapter 5: JAN IMPROVES

Hannah was tired. She glanced across the aisle at Martha and Jonathan. Their eyes were closed, probably lulled to sleep by the steady humming of the jet engines. Sara was feeling awful, suffering from a feverish cold. David's seat was empty. He had gone forward to check on Mom.

By now, all the stewardesses had heard the story. A missionary mother in business class was on her way home, dying of melanoma cancer. Her five children, ages 9 to 19, were seated in economy. Her husband had to remain back in the Philippines to sell their belongings.

Hannah didn't like the worried expression on David's face when he returned to his seat. *"She's been throwing up,"* he told Hannah, *"and still having a hard time breathing. Man, I hope she makes it through the flight."*

"Poor Mom," Hannah thought. She had to use a wheel chair back in Manila, too sick to walk. Before boarding the plane, she threw up what little breakfast she had forced herself to eat. Once in the plane, this would be Mom's first and last chance to enjoy business class on an international flight.

Passengers were served on china plates and ate their meals with wine. But Mom's first look at food had her reaching for the "motion discomfort" bag. Well, at least she could recline her seat.

In a few hours they would land in Detroit, then rush to catch a connecting flight to Fort Worth. Uncle Steve (Mark's brother) would be there to take them to the mission house of Southcliff Baptist Church. And Uncle Wayne (Jan's brother) would be there to help take care of them until Dad came home.

Our New Home

An exciting aspect of our cancer adventure was seeing God's *fingerprints* on unexpected provisions. If these were to be her last days, Jan had prayed for a nice house with a big recliner wide enough to fit her and one child, plus a pleasant neighborhood where the kids could ride bicycles. The Southcliff house had, not one, but two wide recliners. The house had just been newly renovated with a nice kitchen and a big back yard with a covered patio and great climbing trees.

The neighborhood was nice, within easy walking distance to the church. And within a short time, a friend from Birchman Baptist Church gave us a couple of bicycles. What Jan really appreciated were the meals brought over by different families. Not that she could eat much, but she was grateful that she didn't have to worry about food for the kids. Birchman had also given us a "pounding", so we had plenty of canned goods, paper towels, toilet paper, and other such items. In addition, a family had provided their van for us to use.

Jan's younger brother, Wayne, helped the kids get settled, plus entertained them with trips to the park, museums, and a movie. But most of the time, the girls stayed near Mom, making sure she was taken care of, and limiting her visitors. As much as Jan loved to be with people, it quickly drained what little energy she had. As Sara wrote on June 16, 2005:

We are very, very thankful for our patient, understanding friends who've brought food and other things by the house, but haven't stayed to visit long or pressure us to go out. We are still getting over our jet-lag and colds. I'm recovered and so is Martha (she got sick too). Only now Hannah has it. Please pray they'll get well, and that Mom will not catch it. We still don't feel much like going places. I guess we're still grieving our losses.

We are also thankful for the encouraging cards and notes that we are receiving. We're going to get a map so we can mark each location where we know people are praying for us. It means so much!

Soon after their arrival in the States, Jan made a visit to her former oncologist (cancer doctor) in Dallas. He was elated to see her again, but saddened to see her condition. After examining the reports, he reluctantly said that a typical patient in her condition would probably have only a few months of life. The only treatment option he could offer was high-dose interleukin, an extremely toxic chemotherapy that would require several days of ICU confinement. Even then, only about 6% of patients will show some degree of significant remission.

Jan decided to continue the Temadar she had begun in Manila.   She would also continue her glyconutrient supplements.   The oncologist had suggested Jan investigate clinical trial options. These are studies conducted by hospitals or pharmaceutical companies that test disease specific drugs on people with the hope of future FDA approval. However, most trials eliminated patients with brain metastasis. Since the second most common sight for melanoma metastasis, after the lungs, was the brain, Jan would need to schedule an MRI scan of her head.

Meanwhile, back in the Philippines, I was finishing some ministry tasks while supervising the selling of our furniture and appliances. I participated in our Baptist Men's monthly meeting, fellowshipping one last time with my spiritual brothers whom I had seen grow through the years in their relationship with the Lord. I traveled to Roxas City, where Hannah and Martha were born, where we had made our first steps in ministry, where we had planted our first church. With Jan in her present condition, and with me still at high risk for reoccurrence, I figured I was saying my last goodbyes.

The evening before my departure, several church members treated me to a seafood dinner at the beach. While eating shrimp, clams, and local fruits, we watched the evening sun paint the sky orange, then fall gracefully beneath distant waters. Twenty four hours later, I was watching another sunset, but this time from a 747 somewhere over Guam.

Jan's First Website Entries

I arrived back in Fort Worth in time for a Father's Day treat – a special meal prepared by Hannah. It was great to have the entire family around the dinner table again. Jan seemed to be feeling a bit better. Later in the week, after visiting her Dallas oncologist, she wrote her first Caringbridge entry, on June 23, 2005:

My oncologist almost skipped into the room with a big grin on his face. *"I have good news for you! The MRI (brain) is clear – no metastases!"* He was so glad to give me some good news – quite a contrast from 2 weeks ago when he greeted me soberly with how very sorry he was that the cancer had progressed so far. Additional good news is that my lab work looks VERY good – despite 2 rounds of chemotherapy, my blood counts are all normal. My liver functions remain normal also.

I was happy to share with him also that I am feeling better – since Saturday I have not had pain from the spleen, which seems to have diminished some in size. Also, the paralysis in my chin seems to have abated with just the numbness remaining. My various prescriptions seem to be helping with nausea and other problems – and I gained a pound. (Never thought I would rejoice at gaining weight!) We just all felt like dancing!

Please pray for my oncologist, that he would come to understand my faith, my hope, and my trust in God as revealed through His Son Jesus Christ. Another patient has shared with him a book of Scriptures and he wanted to approach the rabbi of their synagogue about having Hebrew Scriptures (Old Testament) verses in a pamphlet form to give to members when they are facing trials. Pray with me that God's Word will not return empty, but will accomplish what God desires. (Isaiah 55: 11)

And yes – Mark is with us – although tired with a cold and exhausted from a whirlwind busy 2 weeks. He filled us in on the sale of our things, crating, goodbye scenes with friends, the departure of the parakeets and Daisy, our younger dachshund as well as the painful good-bye to Duke, our 15-year-old dachshund. Although Duke couldn't see or hear well, he was a faithful mouse and snake catcher up until the end. There was no one to care for him and we felt it too hard for him to adjust to another place, so Mark had the vet come to the house and put him to sleep. He was buried in the empty lot across from our house.

As Mark described the echoes of the empty house, it seemed that Jonathan was hit with the finality of it all. He crawled next to me and wailed, *"It's all gone! I miss Duke and Daisy and our house and I won't ever see them again..."*

I don't know if he relates any of this to future changes in our family, although he and I had a short talk about heaven on Friday while he was waiting for friends to pick him up. I read that children at this age have the greatest emotional upheaval. How thankful I am that you are upholding Jonathan, as well as the other children, in your prayers!

My weight gain may be the result of the seven-course formal dinner meal that Hannah fixed for Mark for Father's Day. This was her final in Home Economics and we all gave her an A+. It was delicious from the cheese ball appetizer to the banana chocolate crème pie – everything made from scratch.

A dear friend from Southcliff Baptist graced us with her presence along with letting us borrow her crystal, silverware, napkin rings, tablecloth, etc. We even put our shoes on! (Those of us who know our Filipino custom know that we don't wear shoes inside the house.)

Now that Mark is here, we have many things to talk about and "settling in" issues to do. I will have 7 days off the chemotherapy, and then resume next week after seeing the Ft. Worth oncologist next Monday.

We enjoyed the Open House on Friday, seeing friends from here in Ft. Worth as well as Burleson, Dallas and even Houston. How truly wealthy we are in friends! So many who are willing to help us, as well as "not yet met" friends at Southcliff waiting to step in when they are needed. And our friends who are reading this website, to keep updated in prayer. Thank you so much. We are so blessed.

But most of all, our loving God. Over and over again, I can only say to people. He is SO GOOD. We see evidence of His mercies to us every day. We can only praise and thank Him. It is a wonderful thing to have the Lord God Almighty, Creator of heaven and earth, to walk beside us through this adventure."

"This is what the LORD says – He who created you, O Jacob, He who formed you, O Israel: 'Fear not, for I have redeemed you; I have called you by name; you are mine. When you pass through the waters, I will be with you. And when you pass through the rivers, they will not sweep over you. When you walk through the fire, you will not be burned... For I am the LORD, your God, the Holy One of Israel, your Savior'" (Isaiah 43:1-3).

These verses from Isaiah became very dear to Jan. They reminded her that she was precious to God, that the fires of suffering would come (not "if" but *"when"* you pass...), and that God Himself would walk with her across every step.

Jan's overall health seemed to be improving, enough for her to write another update a few days later:

The week passed quickly. Mark and I passed each other in the halls as he would sleep during the day and stay awake at night. At our age, and with his cold, you don't fight jet lag – sleep when you can. I am sure he will sleep well tonight as he has been up since 8 pm last night.

This week I have been reminded of the verse in Ecclesiastes 11:1 – *"Cast your bread upon the waters, for after many days you will find it again."* When we left for the Philippines in 1986, we gave our Volkswagen to a new Christian who needed a car. We didn't know that he had been praying (but not really expecting) for a car. (Our car had a new engine, but had been in the family for 15 years). Well, our car is coming back many fold! In addition to the loaner vehicle we have right now, we have an offer of a mini-van, as well as financial assistance on purchasing a second car. Wow!

As with last year, my prayer is that the children will see and REMEMBER the goodness of the Lord and His people. We do not deserve any of this which makes it all the more amazing, but we have learned in the past 2 decades to not stand in the way of what God wants to do and accept what the Lord prompts His people to give. (Difficult for independent minded Texans).

Several have wondered at our financial situation. Let us assure you that the International Mission Board is taking good care of us. We are still on salary and they are paying our medical costs. Of course, all of these expenses are out of what is given to the IMB through Southern Baptists' offering plates. So, thank you Southern Baptists because you are taking care of us! Of course, we have sold everything we owned in the Philippines and if we are unable to return to the field, we will be starting all over here in the U.S.

God tells us to ask for DAILY bread. In the past, I have often wanted to know His 5- year plan, or even 1- year plan, or what about 6 months? Right now, we literally – as we were last year but much, much more so now – will take life one day at a time. And how grateful we are for that.

Yesterday, motivated by a gift certificate to the Christian bookstore AND a sale (irresistible combination -- right, women?), I got out for the first shopping that I have done in months. I had to sit in a wheelchair (just don't have any stamina) but wanted to buy cards for my children. I want to write notes to them for birthdays, graduation, and other significant events in their lives. Lord willing, if this is not my "appointed time", then I will have my cards written years before

I need them. However, if it is my time, God has given me a tremendous peace and acceptance and yes, even anticipation that I know can only come from Him. How wonderful to be given this time to leave these blessings for my children – how many people do you know that slip into eternity through an accident or sudden illness without being able to say good-bye to those that they love?

May we join King David, a man after God's own heart, in his prayer in Psalm 39: 4-7:

> *"Show me, O LORD, my life's end*
> *and the number of my days;*
> *Let me know how fleeting is my life.*
> *You have made my days a mere handbreadth;*
> *The span of my years is as nothing before you.*
> *Each man's life is but a breath.*
> *Man is a mere phantom as he goes to and fro:*
> *He bustles about, but only in vain;*
> *He heaps up wealth, not knowing who will get it.*
> *But now, Lord, what do I look for?*
> *My hope is in you."*

Thank you for your love and support! To God be the glory forever and ever, amen!

During this time, we experienced more of God's *fingerprints* – evidences of Him walking with us through our cancer adventure. One of the biggest was in His provision of two cars. A gift from the church of a former Philippine missionary provided us with an economical compact car. Another generous gift from a former MK (now an officer in the army) enabled us to purchase a van, big enough for the whole family.

The wife of a dentist in Dallas gave Jan a laptop computer. Another friend gave us a DVD player. Southcliff Baptist Church was providing Jonathan and Martha with free participation in their summer camp.

Another *fingerprint* was God's provision of a mission house for 2006. The Southcliff house was available only until the end of December. Less than a mile away, the mission house of Wedgwood Baptist Church would be available for us to move into the first of January. It was just a few blocks away from the house of Doug and Selah Helms, the children's legal guardians.

Prior to leaving the Philippines, Sara had taken an art class and showed great talent. When we arrived in the States, we prayed for a Christian art teacher. The Lord worked through amazing circumstances to lead us to a lady who would tutor Sara for a year. Later in the year, Sara entered an art contest and won first place! It was very rewarding for Jan to see her children make significant achievements.

Jan continued to feel better, though she still had frequent bouts of nausea and fatigue. She spent much of her energy researching clinical trial options. Her criteria would be a trial that didn't require her to travel far from home, that would have few serious side effects, and that would offer a reasonable chance of being effective. While Jan didn't have much hope for a cure, she was willing to participate in an experimental trial, as long as it did not lessen her quality of life or take away time with her family.

In addition to her low-toxic, oral chemotherapy, Jan began visiting another doctor's clinic for weekly IV drips. These were intravenous dosages of various vitamins and minerals that were designed to boost ones immune system. Jan was also extra careful with her diet, avoiding sugar and processed foods.

On a warm Sunday afternoon in mid July, Jan, the kids, and I visited Greenwood Cemetery, the place Jan decided she wanted to be buried. My brother and I had grave sites on either side of my father, whom we buried there in 1979. While we looked at the empty plots on either side of my father, Jan started laughing. The kids and I gave her bewildered looks; of all times and places to be laughing.

Jan composed herself and explained that her brother, Wynn, was out that day looking for land to build a new house. *"My brother is looking at land 'lots', and I'm looking at land 'plots'."*

Well, at least she was feeling better.

Some Glorious Days

That summer, Jan had an important task she wanted to accomplish: to prepare advance birthday, graduation, and wedding cards for each of the children. If she couldn't be with them during these important times, at least she could give them pertinent advice, along with encouragement from the Scriptures.

While Jonathan and Martha were at camp, I was able to finish 31 birthday cards and all the children's wedding cards. I still have 6 more cards to go, as well as graduation and "encouragement" cards.

It was a daunting task at first and strange to write in the "future". But as I sorted the cards, I was reminded of how Hannah, the prophet Samuel's mother, would make him a robe each year and take it to him. There was no post office, phone calls, or email for her to communicate with him, but she could pray. The robe, I believe, was her blessing to him and a visual reminder of her love for him. These cards are my way of leaving a blessing for my children. Also, Proverbs 22:19 says, *"So that your trust may be in the LORD, I teach you today. Have I not written thirty sayings for you, sayings of counsel and knowledge, teaching you true and reliable words?"* (Hey, I wrote more than thirty!).

In each card, I wanted to share a character quality or Bible verse that I felt would be meaningful to them for that year. Of course, I have no way of knowing what they will be facing that year, but God KNOWS what will be happening in their lives at that point (if the Lord tarries!). I trust that He was able to guide me.

I also have cards for right after my "homegoing", as well as 2 months after (which I feel can be a difficult time when the numbness and shock really wears off). These cards will reflect more of my "philosophy" of living and key Scripture that I don't want the children to forget. Lord willing, I hope to get some of this on a videotape also, as suggested to me by Dr. Jerry Rankin, president of the International Mission Board. He felt that my voice would be important, especially to the younger ones, when Satan, our enemy, would try to discourage them in the future.

So, pray for me as I complete these tasks, as well as the mundane ones of planning for the memorial / celebration service, burial, my will, etc.

Some people have interpreted my actions as "giving up", that instead I needed to quit dealing with death and concentrate on getting well. That is not how I feel at ALL! I don't feel that I have given up; I feel that I have been given a wonderful time and opportunity to prepare!

I am feeling so good and friends comment on how good I look! (still fishing for compliments). I certainly am not an invalid; I just don't have the stamina to go out and about. (Although I did drive the car today for the first time to a nearby restaurant so I could have a meal alone with Hannah who just returned from her grandparents).

The spleen has really gone done in size; I have not had any bone pains since we came to the U.S. and the nausea is kept in control with medication. I think I am doing really great and the oncologist yesterday thought so also. Really, when I came to the U.S., in a hurry and flurry because it seemed that things were moving so fast, time looked short. But now, I am sitting at the computer and typing and can't possibly believe that I have widespread cancer.

This past week at a doctor's office as I was sharing with another patient all that God was doing, she said, *"Well, what is going to happen to you? I mean, do you think God is healing you? How do you handle the uncertainty?"* I told her that God has not given me a sense of direction about my future, about whether this year will be my homegoing or if I will be healed. I am completely confident that He can heal me. I daily reaffirm that *"my times are in His hands"* (Psalm 31:15) and He knows the plans that He has for me (Jeremiah 29: 11). He is on His throne and He does what pleases Him.

I do know that I have tasks to do at this time as I shared above. I am also passing my "duties" on to Mark as he is learning to be "Mr. Mom." I feel that

I need to do this, at least for a season in my life (hey moms! I am taking a vacation! Can you rejoice with me?). I am being freed from responsibilities to just ENJOY each day. Fun! Is God healing me or giving me the strength to do what I need to do at this time?

I don't know, but I do know that we are incredibly blessed – and that word in Scripture can also mean "happy." In John 20:29, Jesus says, *"Blessed are those who have not seen and yet have believed."* We have not seen heaven, but we have many promises in God's Word about heaven – we believe! We are blessed! What a gift, what an assurance, what a comfort!

God truly is answering your prayers for me. Maybe you have prayed Romans 15:13 for us as I know several friends have prayed: *"May the God of hope fill you with ALL joy and peace as you trust in Him, so that you may overflow with hope."* Amen! That is where we are at – filled with joy and peace and overflowing with hope. Hallelujah! Rejoice with us at the goodness of the Lord!

Although Jan had gone through menopause, she began to have some unexplained bleeding during the month of June, sometimes quite heavy. Her doctor found a uteral polyp which he biopsied. The July 27 pathology report found that the polyp was positive for metastatic melanoma. But Jan was feeling so much better that she didn't even mention this new cancer spot in her journal the next day:

It has been a FANTASTIC week! I cannot believe how good I feel. My spleen can barely be felt. I took no nausea medicine for 5 days until I started another round of the oral chemotherapy yesterday. I drove the car 4 times (okay, short distances only) and was out of the house every day (okay, so 4 of those days were to doctors' offices…). I met a goal which was to attend the wedding of one of our Philippine missionary kids. It was a long day but we did it!

I am feeling so good, that Tuesday we took a little road trip a few hours east to the East Texas Oil Museum.

I visited there in 1995 and have wanted to take the children. We overnighted so there wasn't too much driving in 1 day. We had a great time and I walked through the museum like I used to 2 years ago before all of this cancer started!...

It is interesting in that I am feeling so good, the spleen (my visible reminder of cancer) is barely palpable, and yet my liver enzymes have doubled in the last month – which my oncologist says is an indicator of the cancer progressing. God is in control!

Again, we feel so incredibly blessed to have so many people around the world praying for us. Sometimes, we ourselves wonder how to pray. I believe we are to pray for healing (James 5) and yet we do not demand healing or expect God to heal just because we ask – just as Jesus prayed for the cup to pass from Him, *"not as I will, but as you will"* (Matthew 26:39). Rusty Freeman in his book Journey into Day said "even if by some miracle we would be healed, we would be healed only to die again."

Bill Bright (founder of Campus Crusade) faced that same decision when he was told that he had a terminal disease. In his book The Journey Home (great book!), he says *"I can accept the life sentence of terminal disease as permitted by God, but I also believe God is able to heal, and by faith, I believed I should have an attitude to seek His healing... Why do some receive healing and other die? Our sovereign God has the answer in His will and His timing, and I trust Him. His ways are perfect... I am praying to be healed that my Lord would be glorified, but I am also ready to go. Mine is a win-win experience."*

I agree. While it makes me sad to think of leaving the children and Mark, I do have the promise of my heavenly home and being with Jesus. I can relate to Paul who said, *"For to me, to live is Christ and to die is gain. If I am to go on living in the body, this will mean fruitful labor for me. Yet what shall I choose? I do not know! I am torn between the two: I desire to depart and be with Christ, which is better by far; but it is more necessary for you that I remain in the body"* (Phil. 1: 21 – 24).

So we just take it day by day – and He is giving me some glorious days!

A Dude Ranch and Smokey Mountains

By early August, Jan was feeling well enough to consider another vacation. I would be taking David back to college in Tennessee in a few weeks and figured it would be a good opportunity for a family vacation in Smokey Mountain National Park. But Jan's fatigue and occasional nausea demanded she stay closer to home. On August 7, 2005, she wrote:

Greetings! I am still continuing to feel great – probably better than I have in over a year since my first surgery.

If you followed the story on Susan Torres (the 26 year old brain damaged woman that was kept on life support for 3 months to give her baby time to develop), you can understand how sneaky melanoma can be. She had had a melanoma removed when she was 17 years old, but was totally unaware of any metastasis until she had the stroke due to brain melanoma.

While I am doing great, I am aware that I also am at high risk for brain metastasis. (Since May I have had numbness in my chin/jaw that the doctor says is probably a small metastasis on the nerve that goes to that area, perhaps at the base of the skull). So I feel an urgency to get my "tasks" done – then I can just play if the Lord chooses to heal me.

But that doesn't mean that we don't play or have fun now. But maybe some folks think we need to have MORE fun. This past week we received 3 anonymous gifts from 3 different locations – all designated for us to go on a vacation and have FUN.

So we are going to try and do that! We have investigated a DUDE ranch in south Texas and that looks like fun because there are many activities on the ranch – I could rest or participate, depending on how I feel…

Two months ago we would have never dreamed that I would feel up to a vacation. What a great God we serve! And if I didn't have cancer, we wouldn't have been given this opportunity. So we can be thankful. And as always, we are thankful for your support and your prayers.

Now it is time for us to leave for worship. I still cry
when we sing. The first time I did that, Jonathan sat
with his arm around me, then matter of factly asked,
"So, what's the problem?" No problem – it is just that
the words are so real and meaningful, the promise of
heaven is so near, the love of God so evident."

"My Jesus, My Savior, Lord there is none like you. All of
my days I want to praise the wonders of your mighty love.
My comfort, my shelter, tower of refuge and strength, all
that I am, all that I have ever want to praise your name.
I shout for joy at the works of your hand. Forever I'll
love you, forever I'll stand. Nothing compares to the
promise I have in you."

May you enjoy the presence of the almighty God
today in corporate worship!

On August 10, David drove Jan and his siblings to
the dude ranch outside of Kerrville, Texas. I (the introvert)
stayed home for my vacation, and to catch up on some overdue
correspondences. The family enjoyed three days of swimming,
games, and delicious food. The highlights were watching Mom
tumble down a slide, try to paddle a canoe, play ping-pong,
and ride a Texas-sized horse. They all enjoyed the hot tub (no
Bubble Bath).

People were often amazed how this terminally ill lady,
eaten up with cancer, would inevitably find ways to encourage
them. On the way back home, Jan and the kids stopped over
to have lunch with a couple who had done short term mission
work in the Philippines, and were wanting to return. Jan's
warmth and her entertaining personality blessed the couple.
The husband later said, *"While we were saying our goodbyes*
to Jan, I thought 'How can I bless Jan?' Before I could say
anything, Jan looked at me with all sincerity and said, "So how
can we help you get back to the Philippines?" Cancer never
hindered God's love from flowing through Jan.

After they returned, I took David, Martha, and Jonathan
on a long trip to the Smokey Mountains in Tennessee. I wrote
about our trip in the September 2 journal entry:

The four of us were strolling along the trail, recalling the beauty of the day, when the black bear crossed in front of us. Barely fifteen yards away, he closed the distance to ten as he sniffed at us with his nose in the air. Most likely it was the odor of our seven miles of hiking that caused him to loose interest. He grunted *"peew"* in bear language, turned, and rambled toward distant trees.

Then there was the 'tubing' experience. Sixteen dollars bought us four round tubes which we took two miles up The Deep River. That's where the adventure began. Sitting in our tubes in cold, cold water, the river took us through a series of rapids and short waterfalls. Our 'team' suffered crashes, spill-overs, and bruises. But upon reaching the end, Jonathan exclaimed, *"This is the best fun I've ever had!"*

But that fun was gone a few days later when we had to say *"Goodbye"* to David. Jonathan and Martha clung to David on the porch of his college dorm, not wanting to let go of their beloved big brother. Tears still streamed from Jonathan's eyes twenty minutes later as we drove down the interstate leading out of Jackson, Tennessee.

Well, we're back in Fort Worth now. That means school work, doctor appointments, house management, and meals to prepare. Jan continues to feel pretty good as long as she gets her two-hour nap each day. She has been accepted into a clinical vaccine trial at Baylor Medical in Dallas. It's a biological, non-chemo trial that stimulates the patients own blood to fight the cancer cells. As in most clinical trials, the odds of success are not high, but, because of its nearly zero toxic level, we felt it was the best option available.

We continue to be blessed by the generosity of many people. Thank you very, very much for remembering us in your prayers. The Lord has truly been good to us. We know that whatever direction our lives take, He will be there ready for us before we even get there.

Here is Jan's journal entry for September 10, 2005. She had already been accepted into the dendridic cell clinical trial, but there were delays in getting the vaccine. Observe how Jan works through her frustrations:

> Would you let me just share about how I process things and you will know how to pray for me? I like life fairly orderly and routine; I am a "list" person. I have my calendar, school plans, etc. (okay, I hear some of ya'll laughing already as you think of how unpredictable our life has become this past year). I realize that in the past one and a half years as we have gone through our cancer "adventure", that the area of my greatest challenge is schedules. I practically had a meltdown last year at MDAnderson Cancer Center when, after waiting 3 weeks to get results back from my surgeries and pathology reports, I was told that I couldn't see the oncologist for another 3 weeks. My family was waiting in the Philippines to know what direction our lives were going to take. When was I going to see them again? More waiting?
>
> However, when I got home that night and went into the Lord's presence to reflect on the day and my experience, I read Psalm 20: *"Now I know that the Lord saves his anointed; He answers him from His holy heaven with the saving power of his right hand. Some trust in chariots and some in horses, but we trust in the name of the LORD our God. They are brought to their knees and fall, but we rise up and stand firm."* I recorded in my journal, *"Lord, are you wanting me to see that healing comes through you – and not to put my hope and trust in what the oncologist says?"* And I rested and trusted in God's timing to see the oncologist.
>
> Of course, God knew the bigger picture because at that very time in the Philippines, Mark was on his way to the doctor – and on his way to discovering the large kidney tumor that would bring the family back to the U.S. within the next 2 weeks. So, seeing the oncologist wasn't so relevant to our family's situation!
>
> Once again I find myself faced with my scheduling nemesis – this time regarding the clinical trial in Dallas. The research doctor, my oncologist and I had anticipated starting the trial as soon as possible which would be 30 days after being off chemotherapy. At this point, due to

scheduling that I don't understand, the initial screening won't even take place until this Tuesday, September 13, which is 4 weeks after my last round of chemotherapy. Then we must wait on the lab results to be returned, which is taking 9+ days, before scheduling the first part of the trial, which is called the aphaeresis. Aphaeresis is a 3 – 4 hour procedure that will remove dendritic cells from my blood.

Since this procedure is not done on Fridays, we then are looking at the week of September 26, or 6 weeks after my chemotherapy. Then it will take an additional 2+ weeks to develop the vaccine (the research nurse says that this is an optimistic time frame). So we are facing 2 months after stopping the chemotherapy before even getting the first dose of the vaccine. (And as it is a vaccine, it will not have an immediate result. The antigens in the vaccine will hopefully stimulate my immune system to fight the cancer – and this can take some time).

On the one hand, based on how I felt in May with the extensive cancer spread as revealed in my scans and the dire prognosis of the doctors (liver metastasis – 3, maybe 4 months), we didn't even think I would be alive in September! God had given me a peace and acceptance about my eventual home-going – and here I am gnashing my teeth at the delay for this trial. (Don't you think God just shakes His head, wondering at us?)

On the other hand, we have made plans to go to my home-place in Virginia at Christmas, and the delay in the trial will make this almost impossible because of the schedule of the injections. (I have a plane ticket for December 15 – I made this reservation as an act of faith when I came to the U.S. in June.) We usually do this every furlough, so it has been 5 years since we have been to Virginia for Christmas.

But you know what? I must come back to basics again – the LORD knows the plans He has for me; *"my times are in His hands"* (Psalm 31: 15); *"He has made everything beautiful in its time"* (Ecclesiastes 3). And so many Scriptures that relate to plans; for example – *"In his heart a man plans his course, but the LORD determines his steps"* (Proverbs 16:9).

So, I bring this before you to pray for God's direction, God's perfect timing, God's will in this matter. Pray for the research nurse in this trial, that she would have compassion for the patients with whom she works and that she would find satisfaction in her work (*"This too is from the hand of God"* Eccl. 2:24-25).

It doesn't make any "sense" that I am feeling as good as I am. I really don't think it is just the chemotherapy, as the doctors believe (so then why am I so concerned about being off the chemotherapy?). I believe that, in direct answer to your prayers, God has given me mental clarity and physical stamina to work on the tasks I had set before me (I still have some "good grief" cards to finish and the children's medical histories).

I have no idea what Mark and I's scans will show; we will try and post an update the night of September 20th. (I think we ought to plan a wonderful dinner out – no matter what!) I would not be surprised to find that the cancer is all gone (then I won't even be in the clinical trial because they must have some cancer to measure to see if the vaccine works -- then who cares about the schedule?).

Or it could be that the cancer has progressed, at least in the liver as my last blood work seemed to indicate. Or it could be a mix of some progression, some regression (as in my spleen). Wow! Won't this be fun to find out?

The wonderful thing about all this (thank you for your patience in letting me ramble; as you notice, Mark is a more concise writer) is no matter what, God is on His throne, He is Sovereign -- He reigns! And He acts according to His character. Meditate on the wonderful truths in Psalm 145 tonight and rejoice with me:

> *"I will exalt you, my God the King;*
> *I will praise your name for ever and ever...*
> *Great is the LORD and most worthy of praise...*
> *One generation will commend your works to another.*
>
> *They will tell of your mighty acts...*
> *of the glorious splendor of your majesty...*
> *of the power of your awesome works...*
> *of your great deeds...*

*of the glory of your kingdom ...
of your might...*

*They will CELEBRATE your abundant goodness
and joyfully sing of your righteousness.
The LORD is gracious and compassionate,
slow to anger and rich in love.*

*The LORD is good to all;
 He has compassion on all He has made...
The LORD is faithful to all His promises
and loving toward all He has made.*

*The LORD upholds all those who fall
and lifts up all who are bowed down.
The eyes of all look to you
and you give them their food at the proper time.*

*You open your hand
and satisfy the desires of every living thing...
The LORD is near to all who call on Him...
He hears their cry and saves them."*

Amen and Hallelujah! And as I read this, I prayed that all... will come to understand this loving, faithful, trustworthy God who will answer their cries... He alone is *"worthy to receive glory and honor and power"* (Revelation 4:11).

We love you and thanks for your prayerful support and concern!

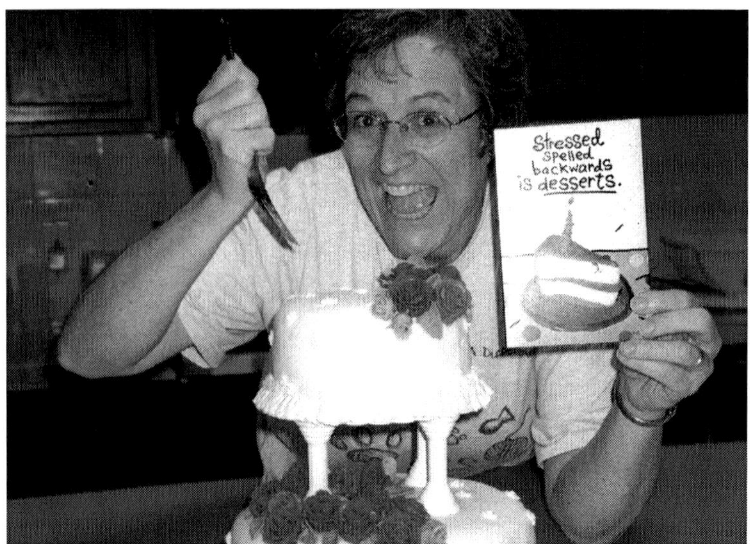

"Stressed spelled backwards is desserts"

Chapter 6: A CHALLENGING AUTUMN

It was a time of unsettling uncertainty. Jan was feeling better, but her cancer was still widespread; prognosis left no room for optimism. The clinical trial offered a little hope, but just a little. My cancer was expected to return anytime.

We had been uprooted from our comfort zone in the Philippines. The children were adjusting again to another new church. What did the future hold? Where would we be in a year from now?

But it was also a time of delightful dependency. For Jan, uncertain days were her chance to draw strength from God's Word, resting on the promises of His daily presence. The children were seeing God send needed provisions through His people. Amidst all these changes, the faithfulness of our Lord, Jesus Christ was the One constant we could all cling to. This was the message of Jan's journal entry on September 20, 2005:

How great is our God! Sing with me, how great is our God! Then all will see, how great, how great is our God!
We sang this in worship Sunday and it has been ringing through my head all week. Scripture repeatedly

tells us that God is great. His word also says that He has great love, great mercy, great compassion, great goodness, great power, great strength. He has done great things, great works, great wonders, and great deeds. He is a great King, the great God. He has a great name. He gives great peace. So, sing with me, "How great is our God!"

Praise our great God with us that Mark's scans are all clear -- everything is normal. The oncologist told him not to bother to come back for another 6 months as long as Mark was feeling well.

I have not yet talked with a doctor but I have a copy of my scan results. There are some new small nodules in various places that are "suspicious for metastases." But the critical area -- the liver -- has not grown. The report says, "lesions in the liver and spleen appear slightly smaller than previously, consistent with metastases which have responded to treatment (i.e. the oral chemotherapy that I was on)." That is great news that in 4 months the cancer has not grown in the liver.

Also good news is that my brain is still "normal", with no evidence of metastasis. (Of course, my brother says that is because cancer cannot grow in a vacuum! Ha! Only a brother can get away with that.) Truly we have a great God!

I am still feeling good -- no nausea, only occasional pain in my arm. I do tire easily and this week have had some 2 naps a day. This Thursday at Baylor University Medical Center in Dallas, I will have a catheter surgically inserted into a vein in my chest. Then next week, in a 3 - 4 hour procedure, they will remove some of my white blood cells that will be used to make my own personalized melanoma vaccine.

Meanwhile, we stay busy with doctors and school and are getting settled into a routine. Jonathan and Martha go to a homeschool co-op on Mondays where they have classes in language arts, science, history and Spanish. The rest of the week they do assignments in those subjects at home, along with their math and reading. Jonathan started soccer on Friday nights with our homeschool support group.

Sara is driving herself to her art and English classes and also takes Hannah sometimes to her PSAT prep,

Algebra 2, and English classes. Hannah has finished her Modern World History course and will start U.S. Government next week (if I get her schedule out). Sara is also taking U.S. Government using a computer program. We look forward to some interesting discussions about politics around the dinner table. David has settled into his third year of classes at Union University in Jackson, Tennessee.

We thank those of you in the "great assembly" who have been faithfully praying for us. We thank God for the tremendous support that we have through Southern Baptists and our International Mission Board. They are covering 100% of my medical expenses.

"It was said among the nations, 'The LORD has done great things for them.' The LORD has done great things for us, and we are filled with joy." (Psalm 126:3). Sing with me, "How great! How great is our God!"

The Clinical Trial

By late September, we were seeing progress in the development of a vaccine for Jan. At Baylor Medical Center in Dallas, Jan had a triple lumen catheter inserted into her chest, providing a port leading directly to her heart. This was in preparation for the aphaeresis procedure a few days later, when, for four hours, Jan's blood was pumped twice through a machine that filtered out some of her dendritic blood cells. These cells would later be mixed with live melanoma cells to develop a vaccine.

Every two days, Jan had to go through a catheter cleaning routine that involved extracting blood through each of the three lumens (or tubes), flushing them with heparin to keep the lines unclogged, and replacing the caps. Hannah, and occasionally me, Sara, or even Jonathan, would assist Jan.

While dendritic cell vaccines had been used before in other clinical trials, this would be the first trial to freeze the vaccine for storage prior to being administered to the patient. Jan was the first melanoma patient accepted into this new phase of the clinical trial. As the first patient, Jan had a unique opportunity. She explains:

I am now the Number One patient for this clinical trial (i.e. the first patient to receive the vaccine). Because of that, there will be a photo session. The doctor who developed the vaccine may administer it to me, and other doctors and researchers involved in the trial will be there. (As a woman, my first question on hearing this news was, *"Oh! What do you wear to such a photo op?"*)

Remember when I said in a previous Caringbridge that I knew God had something planned in His time? I have been giggling to myself that the result now is that I am the first patient (others had been screened but are not in the trial) and the publicity that goes with that honor. I keep thinking that the Apostle Paul was allowed to speak before kings and I will be before doctors. The television spot that featured this new clinical trial in July ended with the statement, *"We're going to see patients who had no hope who now have hope..."*

But I ALREADY HAVE overflowing hope and it comes from the God of hope who has filled us with all joy and peace by the power of the Holy Spirit (Romans 15:13). We (that's all of us who believe!) are told in 1 Peter 3:15 - *"Always be prepared to give an answer to everyone who asks you to give the reason for the hope that you have. But do this with gentleness and respect."*

Please pray for me on October 10 that I will be prepared with an answer if someone asks me for the hope that I have and that I will *"not worry about what to say or how to say it..."* and that it would not be me speaking, but the Holy Spirit speaking through me (Matthew 10:19-20).

Lord willing, I will be wearing my custom brooch that is being made as a remembrance / memorial (Joshua 4: 6-7) of the "adventure" that we have been on for the last year and a half. It is a circle with flames of fire in the center. Isaiah 43 is inscribed on the front rim and Daniel 3 on the back.

Isaiah 43 says,

> *"This is what the LORD says--*
> *He who created you, O Jacob,*
> *He who formed you, O Israel:*

> *'Fear not, for I have redeemed you;*
> *I have called you by name; you are mine.*
> *When you pass through the waters,*
> *I will be with you;*
> *and when you pass through the rivers,*
> *they will not sweep over you.*
> *When you walk through the fire,*
> *you will not be burned;*
> *the flames will not set you ablaze.*
> *For I am the LORD, your God,*
> *the Holy One of Israel, your Savior."*

Even though we have been passing through flood waters and fire, we believe God's promise that He will be with us. We KNOW and have experienced that HE HAS BEEN with us and will continue to be with us. It is a wonderful thing to have the Lord God Creator of heaven and earth walk beside us through this. We will not be consumed.

Daniel 3 is the story of Shadrach, Meshach and Abed-nego where they told King Nebuchadnezzar, *"We do not need to defend ourselves before you in this matter. If we are thrown into the blazing furnace, the God we serve IS ABLE to save us from it, and He will rescue us from your hand, O king. But even if He does not, we want you to know, O king, that we will not serve your gods or worship the image of gold you have set up.... King Nebuchadnezzar said, "Look! I see four men walking around in the fire, unbound and unharmed, and the fourth looks like a son of the gods.'"*

This deals with the issue of healing. We do not need to defend ourselves ("if you only had enough faith, you would be healed") or defend our God ("how can a good God allow this when you have served him overseas?") in the area of healing. Our God IS ABLE to heal me, if that is His Sovereign will. But we believe He knows what is best, what will bring Him the greatest glory and that is what we desire.

Even if He does not heal, that does not change how we feel about God or our worship of Him. And again, we see that God Himself, in the form of Jesus Christ, was with those three men in the fiery furnace. What comfort His presence and words must have been to them! I am sure that if you talked to them afterwards on what it was like in the furnace, they would have said, "It was worth it all to have God Himself walk with us through it." Amen!

God bless and rejoice with me that we have a God who hears our cries, who rescues us, and walks with us through our trials.

The custom brooch Jan refers to was made from the rings she inherited from her mother, including her mother's wedding ring. The gold was melted down and formed into a one inch square pendant of flame with Scripture references on both sides. As Isaiah 43 refers to God's promised presence when we *"pass through the fire"*, and Daniel 3 tells of God's presence with Daniel's three friends, so the brooch symbolized God's presence with us through the fires of our cancer adventure.

On Monday, October 10, Hannah and I took Jan, with her new brooch, to Dallas for her first vaccine. Hannah had baked a large syringe shaped cake to commemorate the occasion. The organizers of the clinical trial wanted to make a promotional video for the dendritic cell vaccine. We were not sure what to expect, but Jan was prepared. We arrived at 10 in the morning:

The doctor took one look at me perched daintily on the edge of the surgical bed and bellowed, *"Get her in a gown!"* Whereas the entourage of visitors was hustled out of the room so I could change out of my carefully chosen and pressed blue jean jumper (I thought it would be accessible enough). I was given a short hospital gown (not my color!) and told to lie down flat. The doctor pulled the gown up because the injection needed to go in near the joint of the thigh and trunk to be as near to the lymph nodes as possible. So, I didn't need to be concerned about what to wear (my younger brother was right – he said I should wear clean underwear!)

The crowd eagerly watched the doctor load the syringe with 10 cc of MY dendritic cells with melanoma attached. He explained to them and the camera what he was doing and about the vaccine, but I couldn't see or hear because I was lying down. Then he turned to face me and when he unsheathed that 6" long spinal needle I thought it would be best to look away. I found out quickly about the procedure. The needle was inserted into the skin and then threaded up through the skin as far as it would go in. Then as he withdrew the needle, he deposited vaccine along the pathway. The dendritic cells are most active in that area and hopefully the lymph system will pick them up, get them into the lymph nodes and then distribute them throughout the body.

It was a little painful but in those situations, I always remind myself of my criteria for pain and endurance (which is pushing out 12.3 pound Jonathan when he was born).

The interview took place while I was still in my hospital gown on the surgical table. I didn't feel very comfortable and I was supposed to look into the camera on my right side, instead of the man asking questions on my left side. The interview was real short, but I did get to mention that my expectations and trust were in God who had faithfully walked with us through our experience with cancer. I did have my custom "fire" brooch on my jumper (which was lying on a side table...). We will just trust that God can use whatever was said or done for His glory.

I'm sure the communications team appreciated the cake that Hannah made, a jelly roll cake and she decorated it to look like a giant syringe – complete with a foil covered straw for the needle. We figured that such an occasion needed a cake!

This vaccine has been 7 years in the making. An initial clinical trial took place from 1999 – 2004 and the first patient from that trial is still living. The vaccine in this trial has some slight modifications from that trial, but they are hoping to replicate the results from that trial. Their goal is a 15% objective response; that is 15% of patients have either a partial or complete response to the vaccine.

I will go back for 3 more injections, every other

week. Then December 16, they will repeat CT scans to see if the cancer has grown, stabilized, or regressed. If so, then I will receive 3 more "booster" vaccines, a month apart. Then they rescan and evaluate again.

I felt a little feverish and sore on Monday (just like you do when you receive a vaccination) but am feeling fine today! Thank you for your many prayers for me during the procedure.

From the beginning, we didn't have high hopes that the dendritic cell vaccine would lead to a long term remission, much less a cure. The patient Jan refers to in the first trial had only one cancerous lesion in a non-vital organ. Jan's cancer was much more widespread. But again, Jan felt responsible; she wanted to do all she could without exposing herself to toxic side effects that would lessen the quality of her remaining days. She continued to take her glyconutrients and her weekly immune system booster I.V.

Overall, Jan was doing amazingly well. The children were plugging along in their school work. And I was missing my ministry in the Philippines. While I never doubted God's plan for us, I couldn't help but wonder:

In all of this we keep our gaze heavenward, knowing the eyes of our Lord are taking it all in and that He is lovingly orchestrating His plans for us. I am tempted to wonder why we came back to the U.S. when we did, in light of Jan feeling so good these past four months. Could we have not continued the work in the Philippines? So many good things were happening. None of us wanted to leave. But Jan's pain was strong and the prognosis didn't seem to give her much time.

But I have to trust that even those last days in the Philippines were directed by God to get us here in Texas for purposes which are still being carried out and for which we may never know. And that's OK. The beauty in all of this is that we don't have to know His plans in order for us to rest confidently in Him. God loves us, He cares for us moment by moment, and His eternal plans for us are wonderful.

Arm Fracture

It was Monday morning, October 24, 2005. By now we knew the route well. Traffic was always heavy when we made the one hour trek to Baylor Medical Hospital in Dallas. I was driving Jan to the cancer center where she would receive her second vaccine injection. Jan's father, visiting us from Virginia, was with me in the front seat. Jan was trying to rest in the back seat of our little Toyota.

The pain in Jan's upper right arm, the sight of her original skin cancer, had been steadily increasing. An x-ray a week earlier revealed a 1 x 1½ inch lesion in her right humorus, just below her shoulder. The lesion, or tumor, had invaded the cortex of the bone, making Jan at high risk for bone fracture. Jan's Fort Worth oncologist scheduled her for a 13 day series of radiation treatments on the arm with the hope of stopping the tumor growth and lessening the odds of a fracture

But radiation treatments would likely mess up the protocol of the clinical trial, making Jan ineligible to continue in it. What should we do? Should we cancel the radiation treatment in order to stay in the clinical trial, which had a very small but real possibility of disease regression? Or do we leave the trial and take the radiation in order to prevent a fracture and to ease the pain? Or how about surgery to remove the tumor and implant a metal rod to stabilize the bone? Such are the decisions cancer folk have to make.

"Ahhhh!" Jan hollered in pain from the back seat.

"Do you need me to pull over?" I quickly asked.

After a few seconds, Jan straightened up, carefully holding her upper right arm. *"No,"* she whispered in obvious pain, *"just go on."* Her dad looked worried.

A few moments later, Jan was able to say, *"I think I might have done something to my arm."*

"Can you still move it?" I inquired.

"Yes, but lateral movements really hurt."

In retrospect, this was likely the moment Jan's arm fractured, although we didn't know for sure it was fractured until another x-ray nearly two weeks later confirmed it.

We drove on to the cancer center for her vaccine

injection, wondering if they would remove Jan from the trial if she had radiation treatments to her arm. In her October 29 journal entry, Jan shares the results of that visit:

> Truly the heart of the king (or the medical monitor) *"is in the hand of the LORD and like a river, He directs wherever He pleases"* (Proverbs 21:1).
>
> We received approval to do the radiation AND stay in the trial. Monday, we spent some time talking with the oncologist who is over the clinical trial. He explained how important it was to delay the radiation until as late as possible (to give the vaccine time to start working), that since this was an experimental drug and results of mixing it and the radiation were unknown, it could be a safety problem, that it was uncertain if radiation would even work on the melanoma, that if he asked for an exception, it might endanger the clinical trial, he really didn't think they would approve it, etc.
>
> But he would try and talk to the scientific team involved on the trial and if they approved, then he would approach the medical monitor over the trial (a person outside of Baylor that is over not only this trial but other approved trials throughout the U.S.) about getting permission to do radiation on my arm. He said he would get an answer back to me in a few days.
>
> However, he came back in about 30 minutes and said that he had approval for me to do the radiation since it was limited to just that one area on my arm. I was speechless and didn't quite believe what I was hearing.
>
> But then I know that you have been praying and God had prepared the medical monitor with an answer. Of course, I knew you had been praying for me when I woke this past Sunday with such a tremendous sense of well-being, even though there was pain. It is such a blessing to be surrounded by such a great host of brothers and sisters in Christ, encouraging us to run with perseverance the race set before us, fixing our eyes on Jesus, the author and perfecter of our faith (Hebrews 12: 1-2).
>
> So I had 4 treatments of radiation this week, along with a visit to my regular oncologist. I will have 13

more treatments. And I am still in the clinical trial and will return to Dallas for my third vaccine injection on Monday November 7. The pain in the arm actually is worse, but much of that may be due to swelling from the radiation. They said it would probably be the end of next week before we would begin to see any shrinkage of the tumor.

A friend asked me once, *"Are you for real? Are you really handling this the way you come across in your emails and updates?"* Yes, God has given us a tremendous sense of peace through it all, but we are very normal and there still are times when I have an emotional melt-down (lack of rest / sleep and poor nutrition are predisposing factors!). Usually I try to stay home and rest every other day. When I can't do that, it takes a toll on me physically and emotionally. The last 2 weeks I have felt very "fragile" and on edge.

One discouraging night I went to bed with my praise music playing. I woke to a song that I wasn't familiar with. I thought I knew all the songs on the CD (old worship choruses, used to be on the "Praise" series back in the 80's). But I hadn't heard this song. In my fuzzy middle-of-the-night thinking, I wondered if it was really on my CD or it was just God speaking to me personally. I turned on the bedside lamp to look at the CD. It really is there. I hope it ministers to you as it did to me that night.

Your Faithfulness, by Brian Doerksen

"I don't know what this day will bring; will it be disappointing or filled with longed-for things? I don't know what tomorrow holds; still I know, I can trust Your faithfulness.

I don't know if these clouds mean rain; if they do, will they pour down blessing or pain? I don't know what the future holds; still I know I can trust Your faithfulness.

Chorus: Certain as the rivers reach the sea, certain as the sunrise in the east, I can rest in Your faithfulness. Surer than a mother's tender love, surer than the stars still shine above, I can rest in Your faithfulness.

I don't know how or when I'll die; will it be a thief, or will

I have a chance to say goodbye? I don't know how much time is left; but in the end, I will know Your faithfulness.

When darkness overwhelms my soul, when thoughts are storms of doubt, still I trust You are always faithful, always faithful."

(Songs 4 worship "Tranquility" CD; Integrity Music)

"Great is His love toward us, and the faithfulness of the LORD endures forever. Praise the LORD" (Psalm 117:2).

Surgery

Despite the radiation treatments, the pain in Jan's arm continued to increase. The radiation oncologist suggested she give the radiation treatments a chance to work, but Jan was convinced it had already fractured.

November 7 was my birthday and I wrote the next journal entry:

Hey, it's my birt'day! Today I entered the lower 48. This morning, Jan and I enjoyed a romantic visit to the radiology department at the Cancer Center. My lunchtime was spent in the extravagant Baylor Hospital, picking up Jan's radiology report. In the afternoon, just the two of us traveled to Dallas for front row seats at the Medical Research Center where Jan received her third vaccine in the Melanoma clinical trial. Tonight I am preparing meals and checking schoolwork. But hey, I don't mind a bit. I'm glad I'm still able to help out where I can.

And Jan needs the help. Last Friday evening, Jan's pain in her right arm sent us to the ER for an x-ray. Today, the written report basically says that a cancerous tumor has eaten a hole in her upper right arm bone – a pathological fracture. This is what has been causing her intense pain the past two weeks, despite heavy doses of pain medications. So Thursday, the same day she finishes her radiation treatments, we go see an orthopedic oncologist – a bone cancer doctor. He may recommend surgery to replace the fragile bone with a rod. We'll see.

Other than the bone fracture, the cancer doesn't seem to be causing any other immediate problems. The vaccine may be causing the itchy rash over most of her back area. The pain medications require Jan to keep close watch over her eating times. The pain in her arm is beginning to cause her to lose sleep. And my inability to keep track of everything occasionally causes Jan to lose patience (some things medicine just can't fix).

Well, pile all of this information onto a prayer plate that would help us know if we should do the surgery, to delay it, or not do it at all. The people at the pharmacy have gotten to know us pretty well; seems we make a trip there almost daily. We are extremely grateful to the International Mission Board for paying for nearly all of this. Between doctor's visits, pain patches, pharmacy trips, changing bandages, meal preparations, school papers, house cleaning… hey, life is pretty normal. As Dr. James Dobson says, *"Life rarely provides us with more than two weeks of tranquility before something comes along to mess it up."* Yet, we live life believing that when the mess-up comes along, God's hand will be there to guide us through it. He hasn't failed us yet; I expect He never will.

The orthopedic oncologist, looking at Jan's newest x-ray, described the upper arm as *mush.* He recommended immediate surgery to cut out the useless bone and replace it with a rod that would extend from the shoulder to her elbow. Jan's arm movement would be limited, but the pain would go away as it healed.

More decisions to make. Will this surgery eliminate Jan from the clinical trial? Partly because of the radiation treatments, Jan's white blood count was very low and her platelets were at an all time low. What about the typical post-op healing and possible infection, especially since she didn't have any lymph nodes on that side to fight infection? Her arm was already swelling from the radiation treatments. Also, a new MRI of her arm showed developing tumors around her elbow. Would a rod even hold? But Jan's biggest question was whether or not the surgery was worth doing in light of whatever time she had left.

Even with high dosages of morphine, the pain was close to unbearable. So, we made the decision to do the surgery. On Tuesday, November 15, the surgeon cut out 5 inches of *mushy* bone and replaced it with a metal rod. The afternoon of her surgery we received the good news that she was still in the clinical trial. But that did little to ease her pain. For three days in the hospital Jan suffered intense post-operative pain that no medication could remedy. Something wasn't right; the pain should have lessened by now. Jan couldn't sleep. She was hurting badly.

In the next journal entry, I wrote:

While I was staying with Jan in the hospital, I passed this verse: *"It is better to go to a house of mourning than to go to a house of feasting. Because that is the end of every man, and the living take it to heart"* (Ecclesiastes 7:2). With Thanksgiving approaching and *"feasting"* on all of our minds, how could a place of mourning be better than a place of feasting?

As I sat with Jan and *"mourned"* the pain she was going through, as I *"mourned"* the progress of this deadly disease in her body, as I *"mourned"* the likelihood of my cancer coming back, I once again reviewed the truths that have become so dear to us:

I *"take it to heart"* that *"though our outer man is decaying, yet our inner man is being renewed day by day"* (2 Corinthians 4:16).

I *"take it to heart"* that *"when you walk through the fire, you will not be scorched, nor will the flame burn you. For I am the Lord your God, the Holy One of Israel, your Savior"* (Isaiah 43: 2-3).

I *"take it to heart"* that *"no eye has seen, no ear has heard, no mind has conceived, all that God has prepared for those who love Him"* (1 Corinthians 2:9).

I *"take it to heart"* that the day will soon come when *"He will wipe away every tear from their eyes; and there will be no more death or mourning or crying or pain"* (Revelation 21:4).

I *"take it to heart"* that our *"momentary light*

affliction is producing for us an eternal weight of glory far beyond all comparison" (2 Corinthians 4:17).

As we approach Thanksgiving day (where some heavy feasting is definitely in order) may I not allow the joy of the day overshadow the far greater joy of what I have in Christ, truths that *"a house of feasting"* do not readily offer; truths that sometimes only *"a house of mourning"* can make precious.

Much to Give Thanks For

Let me share with you one of the biggest blessings of our whole cancer adventure, a big *fingerprint* of God. We call her our "resident angel."   Jan and I knew Peggy Hodges while I was on staff at Birchman Baptist Church many years ago. Now she was a member of Wedgwood Baptist Church, whose mission house we would soon move to. The Lord allowed our paths to cross, and Peggy quickly became a dear family friend. She helped us with such needs as driving Jan to appointments and shopping for the children.

Knowing Jan was having surgery, Peggy offered her home to Jan as a quite place where she could rest and recover. God had prompted Peggy to do this. Being a retired oncology nurse, Peggy was the idea person to take care of Jan. So, for over a week, Jan stayed in her house, while me and the kids would make quick trips each day to visit. On the day after Thanksgiving, I wrote:

"Give thanks to the Lord, for He is good, His love endures forever.
Give thanks to the God of gods, His love endures forever.
Give thanks to the Lord of lords, His love endures forever" (Psalm 136).

After a delicious Thanksgiving dinner (provided by dear friends), Jan led the family in remembering those times in our lives when we saw the enduring love of God. We recalled the Lord bringing Jan and me together, the birth of each child, the places we were privileged to minister, and the people He brought into our lives. It was a day to give thanks and to count our many blessings.

Jan has continued to recuperate at the home of Peggy Hodges, where friends have provided plenty of food and care. Jan was able to travel to Dallas last Monday for her vaccine injection. David arrived home yesterday (Wednesday) from college and will return on Sunday. This weekend we will be in Oklahoma to enjoy a reunion of my side of the family. Jan plans to attend, but will have to limit the time she can visit.

Earlier this week, the oncologist revamped Jan's pain medications. For the first time in nearly a month, Jan found some relief from the intense pain in her right arm. But the medications leave her weak and tired, needing lots of rest. Our hope is that her arm will heal to the point she can reduce her pain medicines. An MRI last week on her right arm did reveal some new metastasis forming near her elbow.

Still, Jan knows that these are *"momentary light afflictions"* compared to the *"eternal weight of glory"* that awaits each of us who have placed our hope, our trust, our lives into the loving arms of our Savior, Jesus Christ. May you, too, pause to look back at those evidences of God's presence in your life. For indeed, His love endures forever.

That weekend, with David home for Thanksgiving holiday, we drove to Oklahoma for a reunion of my mother's side of the family. Despite intense pain in her arm, Jan enjoyed visiting with my kinfolk. When we arrived home, a friend had set up a beautiful decorated Christmas tree in our house. Days later, a dear family played Santa Clause and surprised our family with incredible gifts. More blessings – God's *fingerprints*.

Jan began another series of radiation treatments, this time on the lower portion of her arm where new lesions had been detected. The treatments would conclude the day before Jan and I planned to fly to Virginia for Christmas on December 21. The kids would drive on ahead and meet us there. Jan figured this was her last chance to see her home in Virginia. Still, the pain in Jan's arm was unrelenting. It lead Jan to write:

...One thing I have wanted to study is what God's Word says about pain. Of course, the first 2 references to pain are because of Adam and Eve's sin (Genesis 3). Pain is in the world because of sin. The next reference to pain (in my little concordance) is Genesis 6 before the flood. *"The LORD was grieved that He had made man on the earth, and HIS HEART WAS FILLED WITH PAIN."* Doesn't that make you want to weep when you think of God's pain? At creation, everything was good and now God is grieved. That is real pain. My pain can be alleviated with morphine, but those of you who have had loved ones make bad sinful decisions know of that aching heart breaking pain. I can't imagine what God felt...

...But I just rest in His faithfulness, as I shared with you a few weeks ago. He is able to do far more abundantly anything that I could even think or ask. But if He chooses not to, I can trust Him in that decision also. I'm so glad that He is in charge. Again, it is a miracle that I am still here -- next week it will be 7 months since my diagnosis of liver metastasis. And as far as we know, it has still not spread to the brain; another amazing protection of God.

Pray Philippians 1 with me: that *"I will continue to rejoice for I know that through your prayers and the help given by the Spirit of Jesus Christ, what has happened to me will turn out for my deliverance. I eagerly expect and hope that I will in no way be ashamed, but will have SUFFICIENT COURAGE so that now as always Christ will be exalted in my body, whether by life or by death."*

On December 13, 2005, Jan's journal entry told of our travel plans:

The holidays are growing close! David finishes his semester with 2 finals this week. I will have repeat CT scans and MRI of brain done on Thursday, December 15. On Saturday, David will drive the rest of his siblings to my dad's house in southwestern Virginia. (Blue Ridge Mountains! Take me home, country roads!) Please pray for their safe trip! That is the most precious cargo in the world! It is a 10 hour drive.

Monday, we are praying that all of my results will be in as I consult with the clinical trial team at the cancer center in Dallas. Depending on whether my body has responded to the vaccine will determine whether I continue in the trial. I continue to go daily for radiation treatment on the lower portion of my right arm. My last treatment will be on the 20th.

Hannah got her PSAT scores back and we were all pleased with the results. She worked hard but her good scores are also evidence of God taking care of her during these very stressful months. Praise God that, except for cancer, I have stayed healthy while the family has gone through 2 cold viruses. An airplane is the most toxic environment! Pray that I won't get a cold when I fly to Virginia on the 21st. Mark will be going with me. Mark and I were appointed 20 years ago as missionaries with the Southern Baptists International Mission Board. Lord willing, our assistant regional director will present us our pins at my home on the 22nd.

"My soul exalts the Lord, and my spirit has rejoiced in God my Savior" (Luke 1:47). May God's peace be upon you as He is with me.

Just before we left for Virginia, we received Jan's scan results. On December 19, I was pleased to report:

Check out these numbers. Anterior spleen lesion reduced 35%. Posterior spleen lesion reduced 26%. Anterior liver lesion reduced 37%. Nodules in Jan's lungs, breast, and kidney are either stable to slightly decreased in size. No lesions in the brain.

Obviously we and the clinical trial folks were pleased with the results. This is better than what they even expected. Something seems to be working (vaccine, glyconutrients, or Jan's good behavior). But we will give credit to the Lord working through the power of your prayers.

On the negative side, Jan's pain in her right arm continues to persist, requiring her to take large doses of pain medication that leaves her drowsy, sometimes nauseated, and still in some pain. Her oncologists are still puzzled over what is causing this relentless pain. Pray for relief of the pain, or that Jan would further realize God's purposes for it.

Also, the clinical trial authorities waited until today to inform us that Jan must do another aphaeresis (cycling her blood through a centrifuge) tomorrow afternoon - Tuesday, before they will give her another injection of her vaccine. The purpose of this four- hour procedure is to filter out her dendritic cells to make more vaccine. Pray that her port lines will become unclogged so her blood can flow freely.

Tomorrow morning is also Jan's last radiation treatment of her right arm. Assuming all goes well, Jan and I are headed to Virginia Wednesday morning. The kids are already there. Jan's main concern is what to do if her pain increases while in Virginia, away from her doctors here in Ft. Worth. She is scheduled to return to Fort Worth on January 6.

Jan and I have learned that suffering for Christ, whether thru conflict or cancer, is our opportunity to proclaim loudly our undying love and trust in our Lord, Jesus Christ, and to deepen our relationship with Him. Samuel Rutherford said that when he was cast into the cellars of affliction, he remembered that *"the great King always kept his wine there."* Charles Spurgeon said, *"they who dive in the sea of affliction bring up rare pearls."* James Dobson wrote *"faith is like Kodak film; both are best developed in the dark."*

May the Lord find joy in each of us as we lovingly lean on Him in the midst of life's uncertainties.

20 Years of Service

About 50 men and women gathered in the parlor of Vinton Baptist Church, near Jan's home in Virginia. Three representatives from the International Mission Board were there to present Jan and I with our 20 year missionary service pins. We were surprised and honored. During the ceremony, lots of nice words were said about us. We were grateful and humbled. The children even received honorary certificates for their enduring faith under difficult circumstances.

During the rest of Christmas week, Jan and the kids enjoyed home cooked meals and a relaxed time with family and friends. Jan's nausea and her arm pain continued, but at least we had no worries about doctor appointments and hospital visits.

We were once asked if we thought our cancers resulted from environmental exposures during our 20 years in the Philippines. Jan and I had concluded that most likely they were. Melanoma cancer and kidney cancer share similar immunological characteristics. Drugs used to treat one are often used to treat the other. This suggests that their causes may also be similar. Maybe the many years of eating raw, pesticide inundated vegetables caused a few of our cells to mutate into abnormal forms. Maybe the tropical diseases we experienced during our second term weakened our immune systems enough for the first cancer cells to form.

The next question was whether we would have ever gone to the Philippines if we somehow knew it would lead to cancer. Without hesitation, our answer was *yes*. It has been our life's joy to partner with God in redeeming a lost world. Our hearts have been renewed by seeing the Holy Spirit transform lives in faraway places. The character of our children has been strengthened by growing up in a third world culture. Our goal has never been to live a long life, but to use up our life for God's glory. We would obediently exchange a long life in America for a short life in the Philippines if that was our best means to honor the One who gave His life for us and offered us eternity with Him.

Does that mean we have no desire to remain here on earth? Of course not. I think the Lord provides the right balance between heaven and earth. From His revelations in Scripture, to the indwelling of His Holy Spirit, God gives us enough taste of heaven to know it is going to be fantastic! Yet, He created us here with the capacity for ambitions, goals, and dreams. He gave us a parent's heart that wants to see our children grown and established. So it does take a measure of faith in God's sovereignty to override the sad emotions we feel when cancer comes to take us away.

If God had shown us too much of heaven, we might want it sooner than we should. If He had shown us less, we might be plagued with fear and doubt when death looms near.

This proper balance led Paul to say, *"I do not know which to choose. I am hard-pressed from both directions, having the desire to depart and be with Christ, for that is very much better, yet to remain on in the flesh is more necessary for your sake"* (Philippians 1:24). I think you can also see this same balance in Jan's December 31 entry:

> *Happy Birthday to me!* (number 49);
> *Happy Anniversary to us!* (22 yrs. for Mark and I);
> *Happy New Year to you all!*
>
> Daily I am reminded of God's miracle in allowing me to be here now. What will this new year hold for our family, for your family? None of us know. I think God knows better than to let us know the details and that is why He tells us to ask for DAILY bread. I replay in my mind the words of Brian Doerksen's song Your Faithfulness. "I don't know what the future holds... but I rest in your faithfulness."
>
> When people have asked me about our faith, I have told them that my perspective could be summed up in 2 sentences / questions.
>
> 1. IS GOD REALLY IN CHARGE? I mean, do we really believe that He is sovereign, that He is in control, that nothing happens to us unless it has first passed through His almighty permission, as it did when Satan asked to harass Job?
>
> 2. DO WE BELIEVE THAT GOD IS WHO HE SAYS HE IS? Is He really what He claims to be in Scripture – loving, faithful, merciful, trustworthy, good, etc.? Does He act in accordance with His character?
>
> If so – if He is in control (all powerful) and He is loving (Psalm 62: 11-12), then what is the big deal? It is not that we have a great faith, but we serve a great God. We are SURE of what we hope for and CERTAIN of what we do not see – a Scriptural definition of faith (Hebrews 11:1). There is nothing special about us; we

have just chosen to believe in God and in His Word as our authority to guide us and teach us.

I like what Gracia Burnham (kidnapped by terrorists in the Philippines) said in her second book To Fly Again. *"The times when life seems unmanageable to us are the times when we find out that God is truly good"* (Psalm 100:5). Honestly, changes are scary. Yes, I get rattled at times. But I come back to His promise that God does not give us anymore than we can handle with Him.

Thank you for your prayers for our travel to Virginia. I have had a wonderful restful time here with my dad and "second" mom. She has had quite a load cooking for the 6 – 7 of us for 2 weeks – and dealing with all of our peculiar food needs. She really has a servant's heart and is the best grandmother my kids could ask for!

Pray for the children as they travel back to Texas on Monday January 2 and Tuesday January 3 (a 20 hour road trip). Twenty-year old David is the driver and on the way to Virginia, our newest driver Sara shared some of the road time. Pray for safe travel – what a precious cargo! I will fly back on Friday January 6. Pray for my time here with my parents to be a special time together.

I already have 5 doctor appointments when I return to Texas. The research doctor for our clinical trial wants me to consider removing my spleen, as it is the area most filled with cancer. Also, we are still waiting to hear from MD Anderson in case I need to have a consult there. I will have another CT scan before my next vaccine on January 16.

I had already returned to Fort Worth. My task was to finish packing our belongings, transfer them to the Wedgwood mission house, and be moved out of the Southcliff house by the first of January. But while I packed, a greater concern occupied my thoughts. For over a month, my right shoulder had been bothering me. In mid-December, I began noticing some mild pain in my left elbow. While in Virginia, I had periods of nausea. Hmmm, I felt sure my cancer had returned.

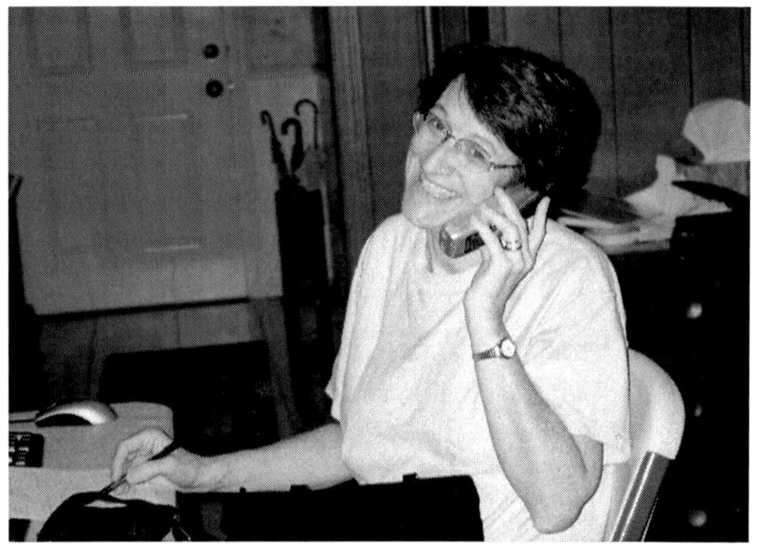

Keeping in touch - spring of 2006

Chapter 7: AN EMOTIONAL ROLLERCOASTER

"I have full confidence in both of you to raise the kids," I told Doug and Selah as I sat across from them in the restaurant booth, *"and to provide them a secure home. You know I love my kids and if it was my choice, I would..."* I had to stop. Tears in my eyes and a lump in my throat wouldn't let me finish the sentence.

Doug and Selah gave me comforting words as we talked about each of the children. We discussed financial issues and about how my children would make the transition to their family. Jan had called me earlier in the morning from Virginia, her arm throbbing and her nausea returning. The odds of Jan surviving her cancer were still very slim. I had scheduled bone and CT scans for later that week, but nausea and arm pains led me to conclude that my cancer had returned.

So, on this day after Christmas, it was time to talk about the details of what would happen to the children. Legally, Doug and Selah would be the children's guardians. But Jan and I wanted them to be more than that. We wanted them, in our absence, to be the children's parents, to raise them as they would their own children, to teach them the Scriptures, and to model the love of Jesus. The success they had in raising their own four children gave Jan and me assurance that we could entrust our children to them.

Still, it was hard to talk about. But underlying my grief in leaving the children was a reassuring peace that God would give added grace to each one of my children in the absence of Jan and me. *"The Lord...sustains the fatherless"* (Psalm 146:9). He Himself is *"a father to the fatherless"* (Psalm 68:5).   Plus, I had full confidence that Doug and Selah would raise them with the same values that Jan and I had sought to instill.

People would often want to encourage us by saying things like, *"You must take care of yourself because your children need you."* While we appreciated their affirmation, the truth is that the Lord, Jesus Christ, is the only person no one can successfully live without. Of course Jan and I wanted to parent our children. But if the Lord permitted our cancers to return, we had confidence in the Lord to provide for our children's needs. After all, they belong to Him, not us. We are merely His stewards of them.

We are to take care of our bodies, not primarily for our children's sake, but for the Lord's sake, for we are temples of the Holy Spirit (1 Corinthians 6: 19), created for a relationship with Him, and commissioned to do His Kingdom work.

Another House

With David and Sara driving, the children returned from Virginia, on January 2, 2006, in time to help me move our belongings into the Wedgwood Baptist Church mission house. We had to decide who would sleep where, what would be put in which drawers, and on which shelves to place our many books. Jan arrived a few days later, in time to go with me to my oncologist appointment.

Jan and I were talking about my cancer when the doctor came in.

"Well, Mark, I tried to call you yesterday because I could tell from the letter you sent me that you seemed to think

your cancer was back. But according to these scans, you are still clear! Your cancer is still in remission."

Jan clapped and let out a cheer. It was one time in my life when I was glad to be proven wrong. Jan was relieved that we still had only one cancer patient to worry about. Doug and Selah welcomed the news, too. Guess I would have to wait a while longer for the golden streets and jeweled mansion. Was I a bit disappointed?

Though moving into another house taxed our strength and emotions, we were grateful to Southern Baptists who ministered to us by providing a fully furnished, comfortable home. On January 9, I wrote:

I hope your new year is off to a good start. We have appreciated Southcliff Baptist Church for allowing us the use of their mission house for these past seven months. This church family has ministered to us in a variety of ways and we are deeply grateful. They have another missionary family scheduled to move into the house later this month.

We have now transferred to the mission house of Wedgwood Baptist Church, who has generously provided this home for us for 2006. It is located only 3 blocks away from Doug and Selah Helms – our children's godparents, should that need arise. We are in the process of unpacking, sorting, and arranging our stuff – a process not unfamiliar to us. It's nice having David around for the month of January. The other youngins have reluctantly resumed their studies.

Jan returned from Virginia last week, well rested and ready to go. Well, so she thought. She overworked herself the first couple of days and realized that she still has a physical battle going on within that requires her to get lots of rest. We have a mess of doctor appointments this week, including a CT scan this Friday. We still need your prayers about whether or not to take the doctor's advice about removing Jan's spleen in order to lesson the vaccine's cancer-fighting load.

The whole month of December, I was having symptoms that made me think my cancer had returned. But a bone and CT scan showed that I'm still clear.

My ailment is probably a combination of acid reflux (causing mild nausea) and strained tendons in my arms (maybe from my workouts at the YMCA). Still, I was grateful for the peace the Lord gave me as I faced uncertain days. As Jan and I have said before, it is our commitment and joy to make Christ known in any way we can, whether in sickness or in health, for however many days He provides. May this be a commitment for each of us in this new year.

During the next ten days, we pressed on with the task of settling into the mission house. Jan's lack of strength made it especially hard for her to prepare her "nest". There were school supplies, books, clothes, and dishes to organize. Adding to the challenge were daily doctor appointments and hospital visits. Plus, Jan had a mountain of post-Christmas correspondence to catch up on. She explained:

Greetings! Thanks for our faithful prayer supporters who are asking what's up with us! I enjoy reading your notes and wish I could respond to each one personally. But when I read them, I visualize your face (if I have met you), smile as I remember you, and praise God for your love and care. It is SO GOOD to hear from each of you. I will have to admit to being most thrilled to hear from our dear Filipino friends with whom we spent so much of our life. Pinalangga kamo sa amon. Pigaw pa gid ang akon pagsulatl, indi bala?

As you have noted, I have not written much lately. Today was my first day back NOT to go to a medical facility. Yes, I had a LONG nap. So, after 6 doctor visits, CT scans, MRI, blood work and another vaccine injection, I can report that the good news is that there has been NO CHANGE IN THE TUMORS since the December scans. Of course, it would have been exciting to have had some shrinkage like we did in the December scans, but we were surprised to have had shrinkage at that point. So basically, I am still on target for the vaccine. My liver enzymes have all remained in the normal range where they were in December. YEAH!

A different radiologist read these scans than the previous ones and he was more detailed. Not surprising was his recording of other small areas (less than a centimeter) of possible cancer in the BONES in the sternum, collarbone (I have a lump there that was growing back in September) and several vertebrae in the spine. (The spine is usually the first place of bone metastases and the area where fracture can cause the most problems.) None of these areas have changed much since September and there are no fractures. There is a tumor in my uterus that I knew about from a biopsy in July.

I had my 6th VACCINE on Monday the 16th. With each vaccine, I have had increased localized reaction. Remember when your children got their "baby" shots? I run a slight fever, have redness, swelling and itching at each of the 3 injection sites. It is painful to walk for a few days but I still get around!

I had an office visit with the SURGEON last week regarding removing the spleen. He felt we should wait on this until at least the set of scans at the end of February. I agree, as I feel I am still getting over my November surgery. (BTW, the extensive prosthesis in my arm does set off the security alarm at the airport).

I am having more reactions with the last round of RADIATION (radiation burn, dryness, tenderness) than I did the first, but the radiation oncologist says that will eventually resolve.

I am having SIDE EFFECTS from the high doses of pain medication. I have tried reducing the long term drug, which means that I take more of the short term. I am feeling very "edgy" and weepy which can be an effect of the meds. For example, when I found out that my favorite bra was discontinued, I cried on the phone to the company representative as I couldn't face going shopping for a new one!

I would love to soak in a bathtub – that would be very relaxing, but I haven't been able to soak in a tub or take a nice hot long shower since my central catheter was implanted in my chest / heart last September (I can't get it wet). The catheter won't be removed until we are absolutely sure it won't be needed again for surgery.

You know how doctor visits go - it takes almost a whole day by the time you wait, wait, and wait some more, as if you had nothing better to do with your life. It is the enemy's way of getting my thoughts off of the ministry of reconciliation that God has given me – it's just now my area is doctor's waiting rooms. Yet, I find myself losing patience, especially when I think of all the things at home screaming for my attention.

Since we have just moved to another mission residence, I am still trying to get my room organized (Mark is working on doing that for the rest of the house, including the garage – where all our "stuff" from the Philippines is now stored). But I am having difficulty thinking and staying focused on my room. And the clutter makes me more weepy!

Also, as the boxes from the Philippines are unloaded, I am finding more of the things that didn't get shipped that I had planned on, things that would just make life a little easier but are not worth the money to replace. Perhaps I am going through a grieving also for our previous orderly and predictable life, home, school and furnishings. I keep reminding myself that it is just stuff and not worth expending my limited physical or emotional energy on.

How minor this is to the many families who have lost everything in wildfires or tsunamis or floods or hurricanes this past year. I was crying out to the Lord through the last 2 Sunday sermons that I could let this go. But the truth is it is there.

Pray for me to recognize when my EMOTIONS are a result of my physical condition and medications or when they are my own selfish choice to walk in the flesh and not in the Spirit. Last Thursday, I was struggling so hard to focus on Philippians 4 and think on what was true, honorable, right, pure, lovely, excellent, and worthy of praise. Yet thoughts of anger were battling my efforts. Guess which won?

The girls said that they also have felt more divisiveness since moving here, although they are now staying in a room twice the size of the one that they were in (they have the master bedroom – and they are so thrilled to have their OWN bathroom!!). This is our

4th house in 2 years. Hannah recognized that we need to pray for the house and the rooms, to tear down any strongholds of the enemy.

You can see that I believe in being honest and open with you – if not, how can you pray for us with understanding? How I value your loving, faithful, prayerful support of our family. What a priceless treasure we have in you – worth much much more than all the stuff and houses.

We are SO WEALTHY compared to those who spend time in pursuit of riches, but don't have friends. We have friends – some whom we know, but some whom we have never met face to face, but who are part of our family in Christ. How good God is to have given us you to walk through this "adventure" together.

A paraphrase of Psalm 71 says this: *"My life is an example to many because you have been my strength and protection. That is why I can never stop praising you; I declare your glory all day long... All day long I will proclaim your saving power for I am overwhelmed by how much you have done for me.... I will tell everyone that you alone are just and GOOD."* Amen! Pray that I will continue to proclaim His praises despite achy legs and sore arms, fuzzy brains or messes!

Adjusting

With the house in reasonable order, we shifted our focus back into the routine of school work. David returned to Union University in Tennessee. I was guiding Sara through her last semester of high school, praying earnestly about what she would do next. Jan helped Hannah plan her studies. Martha and Jonathan were greatly helped by the kindness of some other home schooling moms who had formed a Monday co-op where homework was given for the rest of the week.

We had other activities. With Mom's encouragement, Sara and Hannah signed up for square dancing classes. Martha began a Monday drama class. Jonathan signed up for Tae-kwon-do lessons. I exercised at the YMCA about three times a week, getting oxygen to my lungs and muscles in order to fight any lingering cancer cells.

In late January, someone got the idea of honoring Jan with a "Queen for a Day" party. Actually, it was our way of honoring other ladies who had ministered to us. But Jan played the role of queen. She mentions this in her February 8, 2006 update:

The King is taking good care of his queen" said Helene at my "Queen for a Day" party in January. And all of us present said, "Amen!" My daughters hosted the party for me and decorated with streamers, sashes with "jewels" and crowns – and a queen cake with a doll on top! They invited just a few of the many women who have helped us so much these past eight months with food, housing, prayers, transportation, furniture, etc. I wish we could have invited more, but these already represented 8 churches.

It was so much fun; we need to do it again! Helene made her comment as I was introducing each woman and sharing her contribution to our lives. Ultimately, it is the King that these women serve and represent as they have served our families. Psalm 5 says, *"Listen to my cry for help, my King and my God... Morning by morning I lay my requests before you and WAIT IN EXPECTATION."*

Thank you for your prayers for the children. Hannah celebrated her 16th birthday on Monday. She didn't get a party, but she was treated over the weekend at the home of Don and Phyllis Morris in Knoxville, Tennessee. Mark and Hannah were there to speak at a missions conference of Sevier Heights Baptist Church. This coming July, the church will be sending a team to "our" city of Iloilo, so Mark and Hannah went to share some insights about the Philippines.

There is a bittersweet feeling to talk in churches that are going to the Philippines and to hear reports of their trips. The children said that it hurts to see others go and to hear their reports of "our" friends – and yet it also is affirming and encouraging to see the fruit of our investment. And the children are so glad to see church members from the U.S. going overseas, because they know how a mission trip will change their lives and open their eyes to see more of God's view of a lost world.

Pray that God would guide the girls in their involvement in church here. Since they are not "typical" American teenagers, they don't enjoy many of the activities associated with church – the large bands, music, etc. They don't have many common activities to relate to teenagers about – such as current popular movie stars or singers, sports teams, high school activities, etc.

This is a common feeling of missionary children. They may feel that if they try to become like other teenagers, then they will lose something of who they are as "third culture kids". Pray for them to find their niche where they can use their spiritual gifts. Sara is also working in the nursery and Martha is involved in the puppet ministry with "leadership in training."

Sara and Hannah finished their square dancing lessons; they had so much fun even though they were about a half-century younger than most of the other students. It was good exercise and they would like to continue.

Jonathan asks that you would pray that he would find some God-fearing friends in the neighborhood that would invite him over to their house to play. He is an extrovert and LOVES to be around people. He really misses David, who is back in college. Jonathan also wants to be more diligent in doing his school work. It seems that all of us are having problems getting back on a schedule since the Christmas break!

Peggy has faithfully reserved two days a week to take me to doctor appointments or do shopping for me. When we are together, we redeem the time and have had SUCH FUN at the doctors. Often I have a chance to share my "adventure in cancer" and it has been neat to have Peggy there to add her insights. Last week we had barely sat down when a man started asking questions about adversity. He got it double guns as we peppered him with answers from across the room. And the other patients just had to listen. Another day I came out of 2+ hours getting scans done and several of the other patients in the waiting room wanted to meet me. Peggy had told them my story and it gave me a chance to exalt Jesus. If God can use my experience just to draw one to Him, it is worth it! Pray for seeds that are planted to grow and that seekers would look for a church or another Christian to answer their questions.

While I enjoy these visits, I come home pretty tired. I am back to the point where I was in December, where I can sleep all day except for meals and then be awake for a few good hours in the evening. It is the strangest feeling to just sleep and sleep! I thought it was the pain medicine then, but I have cut back on that. It frustrates me to sleep so much, but if I don't sleep, then I get nauseated and feel ill. Friends encourage me just to go with my body and rest. My pain is under control as long as I take my medicine. People tell me that I am still looking really good!

After I posted the last Caring Bridge, I knew when you were praying for me. I stopped having daily crying episodes and my last major one was when I unpacked our photo albums and said some more "good byes". Also I have gotten some organization – what a joy it was when one of the children asked me where the tape was – and I could tell them! (God is not a god of disorder according to 1 Corinthians 14:33; no wonder clutter can be depressing!) And many members of the Wedgwood choir came over last week to prayerwalk through and around our house just in case the enemy had any strongholds here.

But no matter what, I can CHOOSE to rejoice and praise Him. The Lord inhabits the praises of His people. May our house be a house of praise and rejoicing. We have so very much to be thankful for. Why do I share how I am feeling, even when it shows you my weaknesses? As we were studying in church this past week (we are going through the "one another" passages in the New Testament), we are to share one another's burdens, confess our sins to each other and pray for each other (James 5:13-16).

Also Paul said in 2 Corinthians 1:8 that he did not want the believers in Corinth *"to be uninformed about the hardships we suffered"*. Now we have NO hardships compared to Paul, but as you are our partners in ministry, we want you to know so that you can pray. Paul ends that passage with *"then many will give thanks on our behalf for the gracious favor granted us in answer to the prayers of many."* The result? Praise and thanksgiving to God!

P.S. Please pray Saturday as I share my testimony at the half-time of a basketball game (maximum 5 minutes!!). Monday February 13, I get vaccine injection # 7 – my last injection until June. Tuesday I will see my oncologist and get the results of my bone scan.

In the Bones

Jan's next journal entry was on Saturday, March 18, 2006:

The apostle Paul would start his letters with *"Grace and peace to you from God our Father and the Lord Jesus Christ."* Let's savor that greeting a minute. So much of what unites many of us is our relationship to Jesus Christ – as Savior from our sins and sinful flesh and as Lord / boss / director of our lives.

The Bible tells us that we have been adopted into God's family, He IS our Father, and therefore we are brothers and sisters through Him. That is why I can write to you with such confidence, even though I have never met many of you. We have a bond that goes beyond merely caring for each other; we really are FAMILY.

And thank you dear family, for praying and wondering how I have been doing. I have been waiting on the results of my February 27 CT scans. I didn't get the results until last week and only this past Monday did I have a chance to talk with my oncologist about the findings. The rest of the week I was busy trying to research our next "battle plan."

The good / fantastic / amazing news is that the liver is still stable: "Compared to September 2005, marked improvement of multiple lesions in liver." More good news -- there was some very slight regression in the "target" lesions in the spleen.   Looking at the actual scans, you can tell the difference. The liver will probably be my crucial organ since the brain is still cancer-free!

The confusing information, based on my "normal" bone scan, is the lesions in the BONES (collarbone, breastbone, 8 thoracic vertebrae, 1 lumbar vertebrae and a new area on my pelvic bone). These "osseous (bony) lesions appear to have increased in size... These findings are concerning for progression of osseous metastatic (widespread) disease."   Bone metastases are not usual in melanoma, because melanoma is such a fast growing aggressive cancer. But since I am now 10 months out with cancer spread (actually there was a tiny place on my spleen in an October 2004 CT scan which may have been my first area of metastasis), it has had time to spread to the bones.

I asked my doctor how you can have a "normal" bone scan but have all this show up on the CT scan. Well, CT is more specific than bone. A bone scan shows area of bone repair/ growth; so you could have a negative bone scan if the cancer is growing so fast that it hasn't had time to repair. Hmmm... Is this really progression? Could it be something else?

I realize that the supposedly "good news" from the bone scan – and people's positive reactions to it – raised my expectations for the CT scan. So it took a few days for my emotions to have some downs and for me to refocus on all that God is doing in me and through this. As I have said before, while we pray for healing if this is God's Sovereign will, our hope is not in healing. Our hope is God, who has a bigger picture of what He wants to accomplish through this.

I am no martyr and don't like pain, but God can still work in my life without physical healing. While we are told to pray on all occasions with all kinds of prayers and requests (Ephesians 6:18), Paul's prayers for believers didn't specifically mention physical healing. So I am going to close each update with one of Paul's prayers so that you can also pray that for me.

So, what next? Once there is a diagnosis of spread of cancer in the bones, doctors often use bone strengthening DRUGS (like used in osteoporosis).

However, the clinical trial doctor does not want to introduce any new drugs at this time. Another option would be RADIATION to the pelvic bone, which, unlike the arm, could affect my immune system and possibly may not be compatible with the clinical trial. Also, melanoma is usually resistant to radiation except sometimes in very high dosages. So radiation may not stop the cancer. Radiation itself, because it might weaken the bone, could contribute to the bone breaking. Yet the backbone and pelvis, since they are weight-bearing areas, are much more crucial to treat than the arm.

Again, we need a treatment that will kill the cancer in the whole body, including the bones, instead of trying to patch things up here and there. This is what the clinical trial (dendritic cell vaccine) is trying to do and is having good effect on the internal organs. (As my oncologist said, *"you have gotten a lot of mileage from the vaccine and have done much better than anyone would have expected."* Of course, I told him that God was in control of my healing.)

Right now we will wait until the next set of CT scans on March 27. If my condition is the same or worse, then we will need to decide what to do next. So we continue to PRAY and seek God's wisdom for ourselves and the doctors.

I am looking to see what God's word says about bones and if anything applies to me. Unconfessed sin, envy, and a crushed spirit are all associated with weak or decayed bones. Healthy and strong bones are associated with good news and pleasant words. So many of us are familiar with Proverbs 3: 5-6 but maybe not what comes in the next 2 verses: *"Do not be wise in your own eyes; fear the LORD and shun evil. This will bring health to your body and nourishment to your bones."*

Did you realize that an appetite – a desire to eat – is a gift from God? I lost more weight in February (I'm so sorry to ask prayer about this as so many of you would LOVE to lose weight) – now Hannah and I can share clothes! But I need to keep my weight up as my body battles the cancer cells for nutrition. So pray for an appetite and stable weight.

My doctor also says that the ongoing fatigue is the result of my body battling the cancer (you know the washed out feeling you have after you have had flu? That is from your body's natural interferons fighting the infection). So in a sense the fatigue is a sign that I'm fighting – and that's good.

Now more good news:
• My central line was removed from my chest and I have enjoyed baths and showers again!
• My "power surges" have lessened, thanks to changing my progesterone cream that has expired.
• I am going to camp! You can thank Harris Methodist HEB Hospital who is sponsoring the camp and funds it through donations. I leave March 31 and return April 2. "Amidst the beauty of nature, campers are provided a creative, educational atmosphere of support with a focus on wellness." The staff will include physicians, nurses, social workers, dieticians, physical therapists, radiation therapists, chaplains and cancer survivors. We are staying at Garrett Creek Ranch.
• David has a summer internship job in computer programming. He will be in northern Virginia and we will miss him, but trust that God knows what will be happening this summer. We are already planning a trip back to see him.

"I keep asking that the God of our Lord Jesus Christ, the glorious Father, may give you the Spirit of wisdom and revelation, so that you may KNOW HIM BETTER." (Eph. 1:17).

The camp was a nice break for Jan, away from the pressure of medical decisions. I was driving her home when I noticed she hadn't said anything for several minutes. After I inquired, she explained, *"On Saturday afternoon, they gave us this little project to do. We nailed and glued together a few boards to make a simple little bookshelf. Then someone ran off with my blue paint and I got angry, on the inside, of course.*

"But then I started thinking about why was I angry. It was just a little bookshelf. It didn't have any holes or hooks to

hang it anywhere. And then I realized I didn't even have my own house to hang it in. Everyone else there was talking about where they were going to hang theirs. I didn't have a place. I went back to my room kinda depressed."

And Jan was still a little down. We never had our own home to enjoy. We talked some about our heavenly home, but it didn't comfort Jan. She still didn't have a place to hang her shelf.

Leg Surgery

But what we did have was a family of maturing children whom we were very proud of. With Mom busy doing research and making medical decisions, and with Dad taking Mom to appointments and overseeing the kid's school work, it was encouraging for us to watch the kids step in when needed. Sara took responsibility for washing and folding clothes. She also cooked low-carb meals for herself, Jonathan, and me. Hannah cooked for herself, Mom, and Martha, and helped with kitchen clean up. Martha and Jonathan helped with cleaning, vacuuming, and other household chores.

And occasionally, Sara or Hannah would tap away at the computer with their own journal updates. This was Sara's March 30th entry:

Hello folks, it's been a long time since I last wrote in… but now, I'm writing, due to "A Series of Unfortunate Events". Sorry, I had to say that, since I recently watched that movie. Well, there are several updates. This weekend, on Saturday, April 1st, there are two events.

The first one is Jonathan's 10-mile walk to raise money for a mission project. Please pray that he will be able to go, since he is currently running a 101 fever. The second event on Saturday is the Cotillion for us girls. It's a home-school cotillion. We girls already have our dresses and are planning our hairstyles. It's something we've never done before and we're quite excited. Jonathan was also planning to go, so he will need to be well for that. Please pray that the cotillion will go smoothly…and that there will be plenty of male partners. I know the last part is a rather silly prayer request, but I do believe every girl dreads being left without a partner.

David was here for spring break (18th-26th); we enjoyed his being here with us because we're going to miss him when he's gone for the summer. Pray that he will have another productive couple of weeks at college before he heads off to his internship. We've been trying to make plans to go and visit him while taking a little trip to Washington DC and the northeastern states. However, it seems that our plans are not coming together as well as we would like them to. So pray for guidance for those plans.

Also this weekend, starting tomorrow and ending Sunday, Mom will be at the camp. She's been really looking forward to this! And she hopes she'll be able to minister to those there, and to bring hope to those who have none. However, due to this next unfortunate event, she might be limited at camp. The CT scans came back today, and while the organs appear to be stable, there is a large tumor in her right femur, near the hip joint. Because of the risk of fracture, we need to make decisions regarding radiation and/or surgery to stabilize the bone. There are four doctor appointments next week to help with these decisions. But please pray that nothing happens to her leg while she's at camp.

Thank you again for all of your prayers and your support, not only for Mom, but for all the rest of us. As one pastor wrote, when a family's mother is sick, the rest of the family has to pick up the slack and the family dynamics change. In closing (and in reference to my opening comment), here is a quote from the film "A Series of Unfortunate Events" that seemed fitting to our family situation…

"At times the world can seem an unfriendly and sinister place, but believe us when we say there is much more good in it than bad…And what might seem to be a series of unfortunate events, may, in-fact be the first steps of a journey," Violet Baudelaire.

Jan had been feeling stiffness in her upper right leg for some time, but the February bone scan detected no cancer activity in that leg. Still, it was Jan who persuaded the radiologist to scan below her abdomen to her leg, using the CT machine. That's when the tumor was detected. It was large and advanced, putting Jan at risk for another fracture. Surgery was the only remedy.

Putting events in perspective, Jan wrote on April 5, 2006:

Blessed be Your name, when the sun's shining down on me, when the world's all as it should be, blessed be Your name.

Blessed be Your name, on the road marked with suffering, though there's pain in the offering, blessed be your name.

You give and take away, my heart will choose to say, Lord, blessed be Your name.

This song ran through my mind all week-end as I contemplated the upcoming week. I have read that we can't choose our circumstances, but we can choose our attitude. And we can choose to praise God, even when things are not what we wish they would be.

I wish that I didn't have to have surgery tomorrow. But we are to give thanks in all circumstances and as I have prayed about giving thanks for the surgery, I am thankful. In fact, I can have JOY! I am having surgery because I AM ALIVE! If the melanoma had followed the normal progression, I wouldn't be here.

So I am glad to have surgery because it reminds me that I am alive. And doing really well. I am feeling good, the tumors in the organs are shrinking, my energy level is better. I feel more "up" to having surgery than I have since my last.

I certainly wouldn't choose to have surgery. (When I was processing pre-op at the hospital and entered the "elective surgery" room, I couldn't resist asking the people in the room, *"The sign says elective. Did anyone here really elect to have surgery?"*) I am basically a wimp and not looking forward to the pain, rehab, feeling of helplessness while pushed in the wheelchair

/ helped to the bathroom, etc. My arm has been more painful (swelling due to radiation damage) but will be needed as I use a walker. But I can still praise God for all the new mercies that He showers on us daily – a plush recliner chair to recuperate in, a lamp to brighten my room, friends to help out, my father driving down from Virginia to be with me.

The surgery will be at 10 a.m. at Baylor University Medical Center in Dallas. A rod will be inserted from the top of my femur (thigh bone) through the tumor to the bottom of my femur (at the knee). A smaller rod will be put cross-wise along the top to provide extra stability. The tumor is not removed; I will have to have follow-up radiation to hopefully kill the tumor if the vaccine doesn't get to it eventually. The surgery is to stabilize the leg so that it doesn't break and cause more pain (like my arm did).

Another mercy was God's timing to have me go to camp on the weekend that I found out about my leg; otherwise I would have worked around the house to try and get as many projects taken care of as possible before surgery – and that would have tired me out! As it was, I didn't participate in all the camp activities, but I did enjoy the delicious buffet meals and lots of naps.

The weekend went well for the children also. Jonathan was without fever on Saturday and able to do the marathon and join his sisters at the cotillion. They did group dances like square dancing, contra dancing (Virginia Reel), and dancing in a large circle to lively folk music. The girls said that it was wonderful (although not enough guys to dance every dance). Yet they had invited friends, so some dances they danced with girls as partners, but that was fun too! Then later some of our friends invited them to spend the night with them. They all wore their ball gowns to church the next morning! It was a WONDERFUL weekend!

I ended my last update on March 18 with part of Paul's prayer for the Ephesians. Here is the rest of that prayer. Thank God with me for assuring me of the HOPE to which He has called me (and you too!), *"of the riches of His GLORIOUS INHERITANCE, and of His INCOMPARABLY GREAT POWER for us who believe"*

(1: 18- 19). Pray for the doctors and nurses that I will come in contact with this week, that they too would come to know the wonderful hope that comes with knowing Jesus Christ and being His child.

The surgery went well; no complications. We were dreading a possible repeat of the agonizing pain Jan experienced last year with her arm surgery. But, thankfully, it didn't happen. The pain was minimal and manageable.

I wrote the next journal entry on April 9, 2006:

Hospital stays are no fun. There I was, attempting to sleep on this overused bed-side chair, when, at 10 p.m. a nurse marches in, flips on the light, and checks Jan's blood pressure. An hour later and another nurse, it's medication time. At around 3:30 a.m., the lights come on again and it's time to change the I.V. bag.

Then at 5 a.m., someone whom we haven't seen before wants to know how many times Jan had emptied her bladder. Except, being a foreigner and perhaps of limited vocabulary, he didn't use the word bladder. When blood pressure time came around again at 6 a.m., I gave up trying to sleep.

But hopefully by tomorrow (Monday, the 10th) Jan should be able to check out and move to Peggy's house for a few days of quiet and rest as her leg mends. The surgery went well. A rod was inserted inside her right femur, from her hip to her knee, then a shorter rod attaching her femur to her hip. Kinda like reinforced concrete.

She will probably begin radiation treatments on that leg in about a week. The surgery couldn't get rid of the tumor, only strengthen the leg so the bone wouldn't break. Radiation will hopefully stop the tumor from growing.

The good news is that the tumors in her organs (liver, kidney, uterus, and others) seem to be stable or decreasing in size. Jan has had opportunities to share her trust in the Lord and to be a positive witness to the nurses and hospital personnel.

When Jerusalem was surrounded by the mighty Assyrian army, King Hezekiah told his military officers, *"Be strong and courageous, do not fear or be dismayed...for the one with us is greater than the one with them"* (2 Chronicles 32:7). Knowing that, through your prayers, the Lord is with us every moment along way encourages our hearts daily. But at night time, in the hospital, I wish it was ONLY the Lord who was with us. Oh well...

Recovering

Unfortunately, Jan's post-op leg pain persisted. Since Christmas, Jan had slowly been decreasing her morphine medicine, thankful that she never had any reaction to it. Now, however, she had to increase her dosage to deal with the leg pain. But not even a bum leg was going to keep her away from worship:

Celebrating the RESURRECTION of Jesus is always a highlight of the year for me! How much more meaningful this year's remembrance was to me, when I have come so close to the portals of heaven. *"We were therefore buried with Christ Jesus through baptism into death in order that, just as Christ was raised from the dead through the glory of the Father, we too may live a new life... If we have been united with Him in His death, we will CERTAINLY also be united with Him in His resurrection"* (Romans 6: 4-5).

Celebrating the resurrection is a reminder of the hope that each of us as believers have – that we will live forever in heaven in the presence of God where there is no more death or mourning, or crying or pain.

Yes, I made it to worship at our church that morning, even though I rode in the wheelchair. Sara, Hannah, Martha, and I wore matching spring voile dresses that Judy bought for us. The girls had prepared our traditional meal, supplemented by the wealth of food that the Tuesday Bible study group brought to Peggy's house to feed us.

My leg surgery was a very positive experience, except for the normal hospital interruptions as shared by Mark. The nurses and techs at Baylor University Medical Center in Dallas were very caring. Once we met a Filipino nurse, she invited the rest of the FILIPINOS on duty to our room to hear our story and talk about the Philippines. That is always fun for us! And it was amusing for them to see this hospital-gown clad large white American speaking a Filipino dialect. Sadya gid!

JONATHAN was a bit out of sorts while I was in the hospital and his sisters found it difficult to concentrate on their studies while he was bouncing off the walls. Thankfully the Coleman and Adam families treated Jonathan to a marvelous two days of fun (and his first Easter egg hunt) at the end of last week. And this weekend he is on a retreat with other boys from our church. The girls also found a respite in coming to Peggy's house to study a few nights.

Since this surgery was less extensive than the arm surgery, there was less pain. However, because the tumor had already grown through the bone cortex, I do have pain and it has increased since the surgery. It helps to use the cane to take weight off of that leg. (Before the surgery, the surgeon said he expected me to say that I had so much pain that I would be even unable to get out of bed.

So praise God that I haven't had that much pain – I think due to your prayers!) I have been walking with a limp since January due to tightness / aching in that right muscle as my muscles were trying to stabilize the leg. I should have listened better to my body. I have also started physical therapy for my arm, trying to get my range of motion back so that I can drive the car.

The lesion on my LEFT HIP is not growing, not painful and not in a location that would be easy to fracture, so the radiation oncologist suggests that we just monitor it and not do radiation on it at this time. I will see an orthopedic spinal doctor this week to evaluate the lesions on my VERTEBRAE.

I started RADIATION THERAPY on the entire right thigh bone on Thursday ("my, what a long leg you have!"

said the radiation therapists) and will continue daily treatments for 3 weeks. If it responds to treatment like my arm, then there will be fatigue and lowered blood counts for up to 6 weeks after completing treatment (this could explain my extreme tiredness in January). As the machine buzzes around me, I pray that the radiation beams are weakening and killing the tumor cells – that are in rebellion to God's plan for my body.

While hoping for the best, I realize it may not be wise to plan a family vacation in May. We were hoping to see David settled in his new job in northern Virginia, then tour Washington DC, Gettysburg, Philadelphia, etc. Instead, Mark will take David and show Jonathan and Martha the capital. Pray for DAVID as he must take his final exams during the last week of class (May 8), in order to be at his summer internship by May 15.

SARA and HANNAH will stay here in Ft. Worth and finish their classes and prepare for summer school. Sara is exploring options for a degree in graphic design at our community college. May is a busy month for the older girls – pray for Sara as she takes her AP English exam on May 1 and GED exam on May 16 – 17. Hannah will be taking her SAT exam on May 6. Both the girls will take the community college math placement exam on May 9.

But I still want to take a vacation with the children, so in faith and Lord willing, we are planning a trip for mid-August, after David finishes his internship.

Tomorrow in Sunday School, I will share what the Lord has been teaching our family from Isaiah 43. The adult classes at our church have been studying through Isaiah. How wonderful that although the grass withers and the flowers fade (certainly in Texas!), *"the word of our God stands forever"* (Isaiah 40:8). HIS PROMISES sustain us daily! Hallelujah!

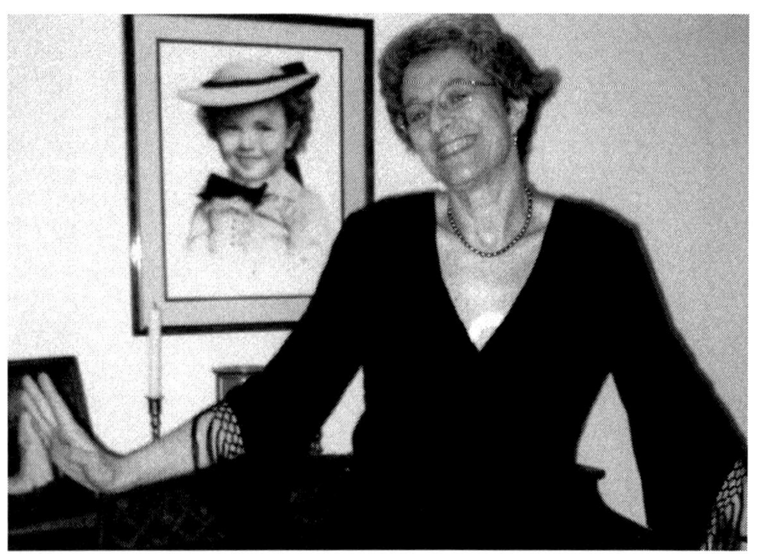

Cancer - the new weight loss program

Chapter 8: STILL A MOM

Jan and I agreed that the most difficult aspect of leaving this world is being separated from our children. Yet, God promises that in heaven there will be no more tears (Revelation 21:4). This is not the place to discuss eschatological (end times) issues, but I'm inclined to believe that when we step out of time and into eternity, somehow our children will already be there, though they will not be children, but matured "saints" of the Lord. I think the reason *"that with the Lord one day is as a thousand years, and a thousand years as one day"* (2 Peter 3:8) is because heaven is not bound by time as we are here.

Well, such thoughts are hard for my time-conscious mind to juggle, but I'm choosing not to worry about being separated from my children. My greater concern is their well being here when they are separated from me. But even then, I rest on the Biblical assurance that God will give them added grace (power) to grow toward maturity. While they must assume responsibility for their own choices, I know the Holy Spirit will to His part to protect them from physical, emotional, and spiritual harm.

As summer drew near, Jan continued to wrestle with health issues. In her next journal entry on May 6, 2006, Jan's growing medical knowledge is apparent. But you will also sense that the children were never far from her thoughts:

Two weeks into RADIATION treatment and the fatigue hits. How wonderful to be able to lay down in the back of the car and let Mark drive me back and forth to doctor appointments. How comforting to be able to crawl into bed when I get home and sleep, sleep, sleep. The days pass quickly with a vague sense of anxiety that nothing gets done but I know that this phase will pass.

I am so thankful that I am not forced to work, like so many who must work through cancer treatments in order to keep their jobs and insurance coverage. The International Mission Board continues to pay our salary and medical expenses.

We are very mindful that each penny that they receive comes from the offering plates of Southern Baptists and represents the tithes and offerings of faithful givers -- maybe even widows on a pension like so many of our prayer warriors.

We are very grateful for this support, while at the same time very aware of how far those funds would go overseas in missions. For years we tried to be good stewards of the Lord's money from the IMB; even now our tendency is to try and conserve -- and wince when we see how expensive the medical bills are. We cannot express enough THANKS for the tremendous support we have through our mission board.

I pray that the Lord will continue to give me opportunities to SHARE with others of the *"hope that is within me"* (1 Peter 3:15). I hope that I was able to give some encouragement to those who heard me in Sunday School and at the high school.

Last June, I had some paralysis in my face and the doctor told me there was a strong probability that the cancer would spread to the brain, causing stroke / paralysis. At that time, I asked people to pray, that if it was God's will -- and knowing that He knows what would be best, that I would be able to speak until He called me home. I believe that the fact that my brain is "clear" is a direct answer to our prayers.

The SPINAL doctor that I saw in Dallas does not do surgery nor handle cancer in the spine. But before we searched for another doctor, he has ordered some tests. I had an MRI of the spine last week which showed some activity at the lumbar 3 vertebrae and at several thoracic vertebrae, which was what showed up on the previous scans for my clinical study.

However, these are not very large and there are no fractures. To get further detail, I had a CT scan of the spine this morning. We will get those results when Mark comes back from D.C. At least now we have a baseline that we can compare and monitor the spine.

Several have wondered why the tumor in the leg was not removed during the surgery in April. When one is diagnosed with "metastatic" (widespread) cancer, the doctors do not try and remove each individual tumor (that's why they did not remove my spleen even though it was quite painful at first, nor the tumor in my uterus although that would have been "easy" to get to).

They rely on a "SYSTEMIC TREATMENT" (a treatment that goes through the whole body) to try and kill all the cancer tumors in their various locations. Right now, the vaccine trial that I am in is considered my systemic treatment and seems to be working well in shrinking tumors in my body.

Even the radiation is considered "palliative" (to reduce the pain without curing) care -- when given in doses long enough to cure cancer, radiation is usually 6 weeks. My radiation is just over 2 weeks in trying to kill the tumor and any cancer cells that were pushed down into the center of the leg by the rod.

I still have some slight pain in the leg and need to use the cane to walk, but it is nothing compared to the PAIN in my arm. Thankfully, I still have narcotics to help with that pain.

As one prayer supporter wrote, with all the jargon that I share, it seems that we are all having a lesson in cancer care! Perhaps this will help you as you pray and as you face such a situation in your own life or church. (Although it does make for long emails...)

That's enough now for me! Thank you again for your prayers for the family. I know that they have been kept secure by your faithfully lifting them up to the throne of grace.

Continue to pray for the older children and their tests (David - final exams week of May 8; Sara and Hannah -- college placement math exams May 9; Sara - GED exam, May 16 - 17). Hannah has an interview for a summer camp job on Wednesday May 10.

A church in Alabama has offered to sponsor Sara and Hannah to attend youth camp with them, but it will conflict with their current plans. We are praying for God's guidance for the summer plans.

Instead of bouncing off the walls, JONATHAN is now bouncing on the trampoline in our backyard thanks to a gift from a Georgia supporter. And this coming Thursday, May 11, is Jonathan's 10th BIRTHDAY. He has invited some friends to join him that day at Six Flags Over Texas (only 30 minutes from our house). Lord willing, I will go there in the late afternoon and bring them a picnic supper.

Then Mark leaves early the next morning with Jonathan and Martha for Tennessee where they will get David. The next day, Saturday May 13, they will have a 15 hour DRIVE from Tennessee to Washington, D.C. to get David settled in for his summer internship.

The day that they are driving to D.C., I will be participating in a "MILES FOR MELANOMA" walk around Bachman Lake in Dallas. Hannah will push my wheelchair and Sara will drive us the starting point. The walk is to raise funds for melanoma research (no new effective therapies developed in the last 30 years) and increase awareness of melanoma (now the fastest growing cancer in the U.S.).

But my personal goal in joining the walk is to celebrate being ALIVE one year after my scans in the Philippines showed the spread of cancer to my liver, spleen, kidney, bones, etc. I have asked my friends to join me so we can sing, laugh, and praise God during that time -- that He has, in His sovereignty, given me a wonderful year.

I rejoice in the extra months that He has given me.

As one friend said, I am in a "win - win" situation. *"For me, to live is Christ and to die is gain"* (Philippians 1:21). All week I have been thinking of the song that we so glibly sing in worship, *"His lovingkindness is better than life"* (from Psalm 63). Do we really believe this?

Rusty Freeman in his book Journey Into Day (Meditations for New Cancer Patients) says that *"sometimes we act as if dying and going to heaven are the most awful things we can think of... Often we make life on earth an idol."* Nothing is better than His love; don't put your hope and trust in things that are temporary.

Thankfully, NOTHING can separate us from the love of God -- not trouble or hardship or persecution or famine or nakedness or danger or sword. *"No in all these things we are MORE THAN CONQUERORS through Him who loved us. For I am convinced that neither death nor life, neither angels nor demons, neither the present nor the future, nor any powers, neither height nor depth, nor anything else in all creation, will be able to separate us from the love of God that is in Christ Jesus our Lord"* (Romans 8: 35-39).

You can pray for me another prayer of Paul for Christians in Ephesians 3: 16-19, and I will pray this for you also: *"I pray that you, being rooted and established in love, may have power, together with all the saints (yep, all of you!), to grasp how wide and long and high and deep is the LOVE of Christ, and to KNOW this love that surpasses knowledge -- that you may be filled to the measure of all the fullness of God."* May we all be filled with the fullness of God and be a sweet aroma of Christ among those who are perishing.

Summer Activities

"Wow!" Martha exclaimed as she stared at the U.S. Constitution and the Declaration of Independence, *"it's right there in front of us."* But Jonathan was more amazed that he was standing in the same National Archives Building seen in the fictional movie, *National Treasure*. Martha and I wanted

to read more of the documents in the Archives Building, but Jonathan was eager to see the Air and Space Museum.

During that third week of May, Martha, Jonathan, and I enjoyed a tour of the U.S. Capitol, a ride up the Washington Monument, a stroll through Mount Vernon, lunch in the Senate Building, a visit to the zoo, a play at the Kennedy Center, a tour of the U.S. Mint, and other D.C. attractions.

David was with us the first day, when we visited the Lincoln Memorial. But then we toured the rest of the week while David started his internship at Datatel, a software developing company in Fairfax, just outside of D.C. The following weekend David was with us while we stayed with a family friend who lives just a few blocks from the White House. It was a delightful vacation and another reminder of how privileged we were to have these opportunities.

We didn't know at the time, but some people were copying and printing out our Caringbrige updates and sending them to prayer supporters in far away places. We were truly humbled and blessed by the loving concern folks were showing this feeble missionary couple. Such blessings were the topic of Jan's May 27 update:

"A FRIEND loves at all times" (Proverbs 17:17). We have been so blessed by the support of friends and our family in Christ, knowing that we are not alone in our *"days of adversity."* In these last 2 years, we can't count the number of times that family and friends have stepped in when we didn't have the strength to go on, just like Israel's battle against the Amalekites in Exodus 17. When Moses' arms became too tired to hold up his staff, his brother Aaron and his friend Hur *"stood on each side, holding up his hands until sunset."* And the victory was won. Moses built an altar and called it The LORD is my Banner. He said, "For hands were lifted up to the throne of the LORD."

While many of you may not be physically here, you are providing strength as you diligently remember us in prayer. You have lifted your hands up to the throne of the LORD, where we *"receive mercy and find grace to help us in our time of need"* (Hebrews 4:16). Almost daily we are encouraged by a note, an email, or a story of someone who is praying for us. A Fort Worth friend who was looking to buy a car on the internet shared our story with a car seller – and found out that the seller had heard of us through the Arkansas Baptist Convention and was already praying for us!

We do not know why God has called forth such a great host of prayer warriors in our behalf, but we humbly thank Him. Perhaps He has a task for us yet to do overseas and He knows that we needed to *"enlarge our tent"*, to *"stretch the tent curtains wide, to lengthen the cords and strengthen the stakes"* (Isaiah 54:2).

And you, our support – and God – are amazing! I have been feeling so good. Those who have seen me (including doctors) say that you just wouldn't believe that I have cancer.

The CT scan shows the lesions in the vertebrae, but again they are small and not changing at this time. I will see the spinal doctor again in 3 months, unless there are any new developments. My leg is feeling so much better as radiation has worked at hopefully stopping the tumor growth. I didn't realize how much it had been bothering me until it stopped hurting so much.

Hannah and I completed the 5K "Miles for Melanoma" walk on May 13. Hannah certainly got her exercise as she pushed me in the wheelchair around the lake, up and down the dikes. Sara manned the water station for the walkers.

It was a great experience and a beautiful day. Us "girls" had a great time as we spent the night in Dallas the day before (early mornings and my drugs don't go together well), enjoyed eating out and being together.

Jonathan's BIRTHDAY on May 11 also had gorgeous weather. The sign at the entrance to Six Flags said, "Park closed to general public for private party." Yep – Jonathan's party. Well, actually it was a special Homeschool Day. I joined Jonathan, Martha and their buddies late in the afternoon and even rode 3 rides with Jonathan (no roller coasters).

He just beamed and beamed with pride. I felt like shouting, *"look at me!"* Afterwards, we had a great picnic supper with cake, candles, and presents at the park picnic tables.

I meant to write that weekend but then – whoosh! – the time flew by. MARK, Jonathan and Martha had a great time on their trip to Washington, D.C. They kept quite a busy schedule and learned a lot! They returned home this past Tuesday.

I thought that I would get so much done on the computer while they were gone, but I have been feeling SO GOOD that instead I went shopping, planted some flowers, tried driving the car okay, as long as I stick to residential areas and no left turns), and started some clean up projects around the house. God knew how I was missing our mission family in the Philippines and in the last week, we were able to visit with 3 of our missionary friends who are in the U.S. on stateside assignment.

DAVID is settled into his apartment / job at Datatel. It will be a learning experience, both at his job and with the other interns, as David is out of the "Christian bubble" that he was in at Union University.

Pray for him as he learns to be in the world, but not of the world, that God would *"protect him from the evil one... sanctify him by the truth / God's word"* and that he would *"have the full measure of Christ's joy within him"* (John 17: 13, 15 – 17).

Another of Paul's prayers for me and for you: *"I thank my God every time I remember you. In all my prayers for all of you, I always pray with joy because of your PARTNERSHIP in the gospel from the first day until now, being confident of this, that He who began a good work in you will carry it on to completion until the day of Christ Jesus"* (Philippians 1:3-6)."

Jan was an energetic woman who would make a list of ten things to do with time enough to do only five. Now it was her health that limited her activities. While most people, like me, would moan and groan in bed with cancer, Jan wanted to be out doing something, regardless of how bad she felt. You'll see this in her June 15, 2006, update:

Paul's prayers in the Epistles center around areas that we would call "spiritual growth" and the advancement of God's kingdom. Colossians 1 contains one of his prayers: *"All over the world this gospel is producing fruit and growing, just as it has been doing among you since the day you heard it and understood God's grace in all its truth."*

Paul closes the prayer by giving thanks to God, *"who has rescued us from the dominion of darkness and brought us into the kingdom of the Son He loves, in whom we have redemption, the forgiveness of sins."*

"Pray for VACATION BIBLE SCHOOLS being held this summer – that many would be rescued from the dominion of darkness and brought into God's kingdom, that the gospel would produce fruit and grow. Let us never become complacent at this annual outreach. Pray for God to work in a mighty way in Ft. Worth this summer!

This week, June 12 – 16, our church hosted four VBSs (called "Power Camps") in four local elementary schools as a way to reach children who might not come to a church building. Pray for the decisions that were made and for follow-up and discipleship.

Everyone in my family participated – Mark as an assistant and Jonathan was a camper. Sara did recreation with the preschoolers, Hannah worked crafts, and Martha led music (the girls did a great job). I worked registration on Monday then got a vicious intestinal bug that kept me out the rest of the week.

In fact, I am so DISCOURAGED tonight! Still wiped out from the flu bug, I feel that I am getting a cold. My immune system may be down because I have slept very little this past week due to an onset of what seems to be restless leg syndrome. It keeps me awake at night and NOTHING resolves the aching / electrical feelings in my legs. My doctors have recommended anti-seizure medicines as the best option but each of these drugs have side-effects. I am crying out to God for wisdom.

I had been feeling SO GOOD that it was incredible, which is why the current malaise is so disheartening. My schedule for the next week is stressful on the body – repeat CT scans tomorrow, Friday June 16. I have my next CANCER VACCINE on Monday June 19 – which leaves me feeling feverish and achy for 3 – 4 days, in addition to swelling / pain and itching on the 3 injection sites on my thighs and left arm.

Next Thursday, I will see my oncologist for a check-up and possibly an infusion for a drug to strengthen the bones—that also makes me feel feverish.

Then on Saturday June 24, I have TICKETS TO FLY with Hannah to Washington, DC to visit David. We are using NWA frequent flyer miles, so we take the "flight less traveled by" – and will fly all over the U.S. before arriving in D.C. almost 9 hours later.

Hannah has a full week planned in D.C., then on July 1 we will drive down to southwest Virginia (ah! "almost heaven -- Blue Ridge Mountains") to visit my parents. We fly back at 6 am on July 4th.

At this time, with the lack of sleep, weak from the flu, sniffles from the cold and a hard week on my body coming up, I am very concerned about how I will make the trip.

Pray first of all that I can sleep. God promises to give sleep to His beloved. Pray that for me! Pray that I wisely know how to take care of myself and that as always, God can still be glorified in the midst of my misery!

And for some praises!! Sara passed the GED with flying colors and is now an official high school graduate. Hannah was pleased with her SAT scores, but continues in her PSAT review course. Let us know how to pray for you also! *"We ask God to fill you with the knowledge of His will through all spiritual wisdom and understanding"* (Colossians 1:9).

Summer plans continued. Jonathan would participate in church activities and spend time with his friends. Martha would be part of her Leadership in Action team traveling to Pineville, Louisiana to help teach in Vacation Bible School. Hannah continued her PSAT prep course. Sara began her first college course at Tarrant County College. David was away at his internship job.

On June 23, Jan shared about her latest scan reports:

Here I am, 13 months from my "poor prognosis" of last May 2005 -- alive and doing remarkably well! I had CT scans and MRI last Friday. There was NO GROWTH in the cancer; everything still left (spleen, lungs, bones) is "small and stable" (unchanged). I am still enrolled in the dendritic cell vaccine clinical trial. We heard that I am the only patient of the original 7 enrolled last fall that has not had any progression (growth) of cancer.

You would think the researchers would ask themselves what makes me different? Well, maybe they don't ask because I keep telling them that God is in control and we have prayer supporters world-wide daily lifting us up to His throne of grace. Thank you!

Monday, June 19, I received my 8th CANCER VACCINE. As anticipated, I was feverish and achy for 3 days, then swollen and itchy at the injection sites. But I'm feeling better now – and packing furiously – we leave for the airport at 4:30 am tomorrow!

Continue to pray for Hannah's and my TRIP TO WASHINGTON, D.C. We will visit with DAVID over this weekend and the July 4th weekend. As a proper finish to Hannah's American Government class, we will have coffee with our senator (and other constituents) on Thursday. Hannah is to be prepared with questions on 3 different topics (yep, I'm grading her on this!).

Pray that I wisely know how to take care of myself and rest when I need to (as a mom, I will push myself for my kids! I hope I can get a little grocery shopping done for David while we are there). I am planning to go out with Hannah in the morning, then return after lunch to my friend's house for a nap.

Hannah will finish the museum on her own and come back on the subway by herself. It's more fun with a companion, but this is the best compromise we could work out. So pray for her safety and direction as she travels.

Between the flu bug and the vaccine, I am still feeling pretty weak. Thank you for praying for my sleep – I am doing better. Apparently, weaning off the morphine may have caused some of the problems with my sleep. So, I'm back on my drugs!

Mark wants me to be sure to add some really good news. We have learned that last year's LOTTIE MOON CHRISTMAS OFFERING for international missions reached a record amount - $137,939,677.59. This shows that Southern Baptists are serious about impacting lives around the world and reaching those people groups that have yet to hear the gospel. It enables our 5,100 colleagues to continue the work that saw more than 459,000 new believers last year and more than 17,000 new churches planted. How our feet ("beautiful feet"?) itch to be back in the Philippines to add to these numbers. Thank you, Southern Baptists, for your faithful giving.

Adventure in D.C.

Hannah stood inconspicuously a block away as the Washington D.C. police drove up. She had just set off the security alarm of an expensive Georgetown row house. Now, Hannah didn't know what to do, but she certainly didn't want David to get caught. Mom couldn't help; she was in a hotel room, recovering from a trip to the hospital emergency room.

Sound exciting? Well, here's the story...

Jan and Hannah arrived in D.C. safely but tired. Jan's former school mate and close friend, Karen, picked them up from the airport and took them to her Georgetown home. The next day, Jan had a severe skin reaction (most likely from the vaccine a few days earlier). She stayed overnight at the hospital, then checked in to a nearby hotel to recover. A subsequent reaction sent her back to the emergency room where she was treated, released, and sent back to the hotel room.

Jan didn't want Hannah to miss seeing the D.C. attractions, so Karen gave Hannah instructions on how to use the D.C. metro subway and trolley buses. Hannah bravely traveled around D.C. that week on her own, during record rainfalls, visiting museums and memorials.

On Friday, Jan called from the hotel and told David to come to Karen's house, where Hannah would meet him and guide him to the hotel. Karen had errands to do. As she left that morning, she routinely programmed her house security alarm.

Later in the afternoon, when Hannah arrived with the house key, she set off the alarm. It was loud! What should she do? She didn't carry a purse. She had no identification explaining who she was. She didn't even know Karen's cell number.

Hannah left the blaring alarm and started walking back to the hotel. Then she thought, *"What if David arrives and then the police show up?"*

Hannah turned back toward the apartment in time to see the police car drive up. There was a pizza boy making a delivery next door. The police questioned him. Poor guy. The customer receiving the pizza explained to the police that the boy had just arrived.

Hannah went back to the hotel room, in time to see Karen rushing out. *"Hannah,"* she said nervously, *"I set my alarm this morning!"*

"I know," Hannah grinned. They returned to the house together where Karen called and explained the situation to the security personnel. And David didn't show up until Saturday morning.

Jan's skin reaction was pretty serious. She returned to the emergency room because the swelling in her throat and mouth hindered her breathing. Fortunately, the swelling had gone down by the time they were scheduled to leave D.C.

While Jan and Hannah were having their adventures in D.C., I was having an adventure of my own back in the oncologist's office:

It's one of those times most cancer patients have to endure – waiting in the doctor's office for the latest scan results. Will the report show that my cancer has returned? How extensive will it be? Is it in the lungs, brain, liver, or all of the above? Ahhhh! Or, will the report show that my cancer is still in remission; not have to worry about it until I sit in this chair again in six months.

"Do not fear, for I am with you; do not anxiously look about you, for I am your God. I will strengthen you, surely I will help you. Surely I will uphold you with my righteous right hand" (Isaiah 41:10). That verse helped me out a lot one night years ago when a bear circled my tent up in Wyoming while alone on a backpacking trip. The bear went away. But this cancer stuff is a different kind of animal.

The doctor comes in with a smile. That's a good sign, I think to myself, or is it? *"So, Mark,"* he asks, *"how are you doing today?"*

Hmmm. He's not saying anything about the scans. Is he avoiding the bad news? Just making small talk to make me feel better? Or, since he's my doctor, maybe he really wants to know how I'm doing. Well, if he would hurry up and tell me the scan reports, I'd feel a lot better. At least I would know.

"By the way," he adds, *"your scans are clear. Looks like you're good for at least another six months"* Ahhhh, relief. Guess I will be around for a while longer. Now I can go ahead and buy some new underwear.

As for Jan, she didn't fare too well while in Washington D.C. A possible reaction from her vaccine caused her to break out in hives and fever that sent her to the emergency room and an overnight stay in the hospital. Our friend, Karen Hamrick, was an outstanding hostess as she did her best to make Jan feel comfortable. So, while Jan spent the week scratching, Hannah spent the week walking. Wading through record rainfalls, Hannah went by herself from government buildings to museums, visiting as many places as she could. Both were able to spend some quality time with David, which was the main purpose of the trip.

Back in Texas, the summer wears on... Home-schooling and square-dancing, eating out and eating in, house work and yard work, doctor appointments and church activities, seems every day on the calendar is penciled in with something. Tomorrow, Hannah travels to Riverbend (our Tarrant County Baptist camp) for her one-month internship. Sara has begun her second summer class at the community college (she got an A in her math class!). Jan and I will be planning next year's school year, grateful for everyday we have with our family. We plan, knowing that things could quickly change for one or both of us. But whatever direction this cancer carries us, we know God will already be there to walk us through it.

Decisions

It was August 4, 2006. David would be home in a few days for a two week break before returning to Tennessee for his last year in college. Hannah would also be home in a few days from her five week job at the Baptist summer camp. Sara was half way through her second summer class and doing well. Martha had a spiritually rewarding experience on the Louisiana mission trip. Jan and I were having to decide what Martha and Jonathan would do for school during the coming year, especially in light of our uncertain health status.

And Jan was having to deal with more medical related decisions:

How glad I am that God knows what is best and we are seeking His wisdom. He is always faithful to guide! But Scripture also tells us that *"wisdom is found in those who take advice"* (Proverbs 13:10). That is why I like to share and receive your advice and prayers.

Pray for the CLINCIAL TRIAL DOCTORS as they make decisions regarding my next vaccine in September. I had hives and fever after my last vaccine, which resulted in a trip to the ER when the swelling went to my face and throat. We don't know if the hives were the direct result of the vaccine or something I was exposed to in D.C.

Because it was a potentially life-threatening reaction, the clinical trial doctors will have to make an appeal to the FDA to keep me on the trial to continue receiving vaccines. Both my allergist and the specialist in autoimmune diseases feel that I should go for the next vaccine as it seems to be controlling the cancer. (We know who is ultimately in control, right?)

I saw the orthopedic surgeon this week as my

RIGHT LEG has been bothering me again. X-ray shows that the tumor has not grown since the surgery and the rod is in good position, so we are not sure what is happening.

The first question that my radiation oncologist asked me, *"What have you been doing?"* Maybe it's all the driving and shopping and cooking! Yep, you won't believe how much I have been able to do. But the leg acting up reminds me that I still need to take care of myself...

Another factor... is HOUSING. Lord willing, we can stay at this Wedgwood house until next May 2007. So we should be able to get almost through the school year in this location. We don't know about housing beyond next May or where we will be. But the Lord knows the answer to that also and He can give us direction in schooling without telling us the total picture.

Mark and I have been so blessed by all the churches that we have stayed at during this chapter in our lives; we know God can do far more abundantly than we could think or ask wherever He takes us.

And most importantly in your prayers – *"Pray for us, too, that God may open a door for our message, so that we may proclaim the mystery of Christ... PRAY THAT I MAY PROCLAIM IT CLEARLY as I should. Be wise in the way you act toward outsiders; make the most of EVERY opportunity. Let your conversation be always full of grace, seasoned with salt, so that you may know how to answer everyone"* (Colossians 4: 3-6). Thank you for your loving support, concern and prayers.

Jan wrote her next update on August 23, 2006, the day after David's 21st birthday...

The allergist, rheumatologist, and clinical trial doctors all agree that I should proceed with the next vaccine on September 11 but with a plan of action in case I have another reaction. The clinical trial doctors submitted their report to the FDA about what happened in June; the FDA is considering whether to allow me to stay on the study. So pray that God will guide whomever at FDA that will be making that decision. I feel comfortable proceeding with the vaccine but know that God can use the FDA's decision to give us direction.

I have had increasing pain and swelling in the right leg and my oncologist has recommended I resume 24 hr morphine. I don't like this and all the different attendant problems that go with it (laxatives, medicine for nausea, dry mouth, etc). No one has given me an explanation of what could be the problem. I was planning on square dancing lessons in September so this leg needs to get in shape!

Thank you for your prayers for school. Jonathan is attending Christian Life Prep; they graciously admitted him even though the registration date was closed (they have never done this before). He goes to school on Tuesday and Thursday and does his homework on the remaining days. Pray for decisions on whether to continue his Tae Kwon Do classes. He proudly passed the test for his yellow belt.

I am still slowly getting curriculum together for Martha; Lord willing, by the first of September, I will have her schedule organized so she can pretty much work on her own. She is showing real diligence and concern for staying caught up. Hannah is home from her summer job and starts her classes this week. She is already feeling overwhelmed; she feels responsible about things in the home and it distracts her from her schoolwork. Pray that she can stay focused on the tasks that God gives her.

A friend has graciously invited Sara to stay with her Monday through Wednesday nights so she won't have so much driving back and forth. Thank you, Lord, for Melinda! We'll move Sara's things this Saturday and she starts class on Monday August 28. That same day, David will leave for Union for his last year of college. We have enjoyed having him home for 2 weeks.

I got really stressed trying to juggle all the homeschooling needs and children's activities -- but after talking to some moms, I realize that it isn't all because I find it difficult to multi-task these days. Other moms in perfectly healthy bodies find it stressful also. Welcome to the busy USA! Life was much more simpler in the Philippines. Pray that I also will focus on what God wants me to do with the time that He has graciously given to me. Paul says in Philippians 3:13 -- *"This one thing I do..."* What one thing has God called me to do, for you to do? As our pastor has said, nothing is as thrilling as sharing Jesus with others. Pray for me to continue to have opportunities to exalt Jesus; He promises that when He is lifted up, He will draw all men to Himself (John 12:32).

Out of the Trial

Jan and I were in the waiting room of her orthopedic oncologist in Dallas when her cell phone rang. From the beginning of her conversation, I could tell it was the Clinical Trial doctor. Jan listened silently, then tears formed in her eyes. A few more sentences and the conversation was over. Jan closed her eyes. She took a deep breath. The FDA had chosen to exclude her from the clinical trial because of her skin reaction in June. Jan leaned over, buried her face in a handkerchief, and cried.

Doctors could treat cancer tumors as they popped up, but without a systemic treatment, there was nothing that could keep the cancer from spreading. But this wasn't why Jan was crying. She felt responsible. The weight of finding another systemic treatment was now on her shoulders. She would have to hit the books, research the internet, call for information, all in an effort to find another clinical trial that would accept her.

I observed that when Jan received bad news, she usually had an initial, negative emotional reaction. It hurt. It was sad. We grieved. But once she got through the emotional response, her spirit would take over. She humbly accepted God's grace and the counsel of His Word. She refocused her faith and renewed her trust. The news was viewed from God's perspective; she saw its potential benefits. She then chose to turn the sadness into praise, as she did in her September 10 update:

All the way my Savior leads me --
What have I to ask beside?
Can I doubt His tender mercy,
who through life has been my Guide?
Heavn'ly peace, divinest comfort,
here by faith in Him to dwell!
For I know, whate'er befall me,
Jesus doeth all things well;
For I know, whate'er befall me,
Jesus doeth all things well.

Some have suggested that we write a book about our adventures. At least I would know now how to start the chapters – with a song and Scripture that God has given me for guidance, reassurance, and comfort at different stages and weeks in the journey.

The above song has been replaying in my head all weekend and on Monday morning, the reading in the devotional Daily Light (wonderful! Pure Scripture) reminded me of God's promise in April 2004 when I first found out about the spread of the cancer – *"He will not be afraid of evil tidings; his heart is steadfast, trusting in the LORD"* (Psalm 112: 7-8) - and other verses on being still and quiet and resting in the Lord.

We got the news on Wednesday that the FDA and the Baylor Institute of Immunological Research made a team decision NOT to continue me in the trial, due to the reaction that I had in June. The decision is "set in stone" and "no options". So I can no longer be treated with the dendritic cell vaccine.

This is disappointing but I come back over and over that we prayed that God would give us direction through the authority over the trial, which is the FDA. That direction was given loud and clearly. We can only trust that God is using this to direct and protect me.

As my oncologist says, I received much benefit from the trial and for that I am grateful. I do regret giving up my status as the Number One patient in the trial. I was enjoying being Number One! Home Interiors, which is the business started by Mary Crowley, a Dallas businesswoman, will be donating all sales of a particular candle this fall to the Mary Crowley Medical Research

Center (where I had my clinical trial).

My story is on the box as a patient that benefited from the Center. I also had an opportunity to share briefly in this month's Mary Crowley MRC newsletter about how God has been with us through this cancer experience. God had me there for His time and for His purpose. Now it is time to move on.

So what is next? Since there is no effective treatment for stage IV metastatic melanoma cancer (cancer that is spread throughout the body), then I need to research other clinical trials. MDAnderson in Houston? National Institutes of Health in Maryland? John Wayne Cancer Center in California? Things to consider -- travel, expenses, time, etc. I do not feel that I need to desperately travel hither and yon in order to stay alive, but I still have responsibilities here and have been encouraged to seek out another trial.

I have an appointment this Wednesday Sept. 13 with one of the developers of the vaccine trial. Since he is familiar with the vaccine and has used it in prior patients, I am seeking his advice on what treatment to follow next. Pray that God will direct him. His nurse has been a tremendous support to me this past year. God knew before we did that I would be out of the trial and has directed the nurse to move to California. We'll miss her!

The next week, September 21 and 22, I will have an appointment at MDAnderson Cancer Center where I had my surgeries in 2004. My options for treatment are much more limited now, due to prior therapies and my autoimmune disease.

But God is not limited! My life is in His hands. It is our desire to glorify Him and for all to know that HE IS IN CONTROL. He has brought me this far for His purposes and, we desire, for His glory. *"This is what God the LORD says – He who created the heavens and stretched them out, who spread out the earth and all that comes out of it, who gives breath to its people, and life to those who walk on it.... I am the LORD; that is my name! I will not give my glory to another or my praise to idols. See, the former things have taken place, and new things I declare"* (Isaiah 42:5, 8-9). Rejoice with us as we anticipate the *"new things"* that God will be doing.

I was enjoying settling into a "new norm" with school, Bible study, shopping and a minimum of doctor appointments. But *"my times are in His hands"* – and I'm not in control. There is so much that I would like to do with and for the children. I am sure most mothers are torn between what they want to do and what they are able to do with the time that they have.

This week is Martha's 13th birthday. The "mother side" of me wants to plan a special party like I would have done in the past with the older children. I also want to help Martha more with her studies (she is trying so hard to catch up from some past deficiencies and get ahead in other areas).

Yet, the "cancer patient" side of me knows that I need to take good physical care of myself, rest, eat right, and allow time to research and plan for these doctor appointments. So the most important thing is for me to daily sit (*"sit still, my daughter"* Ruth 3:18) with the Lord, listening to what He says. (*"Only one thing is needed. Mary has chosen what is better"* Luke 10: 39, 42.)

Pray for Martha to continue to grow in wisdom and stature and favor with God and man. This is the longest time that we have been in a U.S. church, so the first time to be really involved with the youth. We are learning much about the "teen scene." Pray that Martha will keep her priorities right and her focus on the Lord.

One thing that has made this journey so much easier is your support, not only for me, but for the children. Just today I was talking with a prayer warrior who asked about each child by name and about specific needs for each child. Wow! I can hardly remember my own children's names and what a blessing to have someone who hardly knows us except through emails be praying specifically for my children. What assurance this gives me for the future -- *For I know, whate'er befall me, Jesus doeth all things well.*

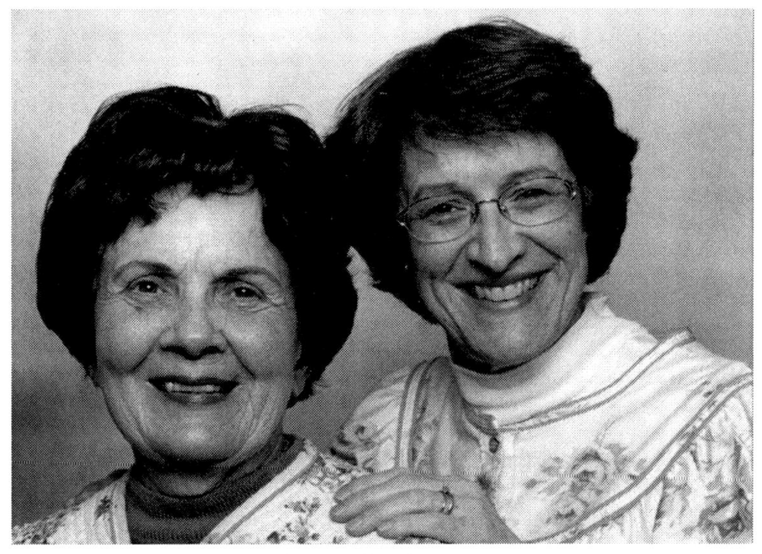
Peggy and Jan in their "grandma" gowns

Chapter 9: A GROWING FAITH

Did God CAUSE Jan's cancer? In our testimonies, both Jan and I say that God "allowed" our cancers, but did not "cause" them. However, in our private talk, we left room for the possibility that God, in His sovereignty, may have caused them. And that was okay.

"If a calamity occurs in a city has not the Lord done it?" (Amos 3:6). *"Who has made man's mouth? Or who makes him dumb or deaf, or seeing or blind? Is it not I, the Lord?"* (Exodus 4:11). *"The One forming light and creating darkness, causing peace and creating calamity; I am the Lord who does all these"* (Isaiah 45:7). Concerning a blind man, Jesus said, *"It was neither that this man sinned, nor his parents; but it was in order that the works of God might be displayed in him"* (John 9:3).

When the storms of life roll in and the winds of adversity blow hard, our natural assumption is that such events are destructive. But remember the illustration of the eagle. Storms bring needed rain that nourishes the ground that supports the life that the eagle feeds upon. Strong winds effortlessly lift the eagle above the harassment of other birds and allows the eagle to see more, to see further, to fly longer, and to fly faster.

We who *"wait for the Lord will gain new strength"* when we *"mount up with wings like eagles..."* (Isaiah 40:31). When we learn to see the benefits of our suffering, then it doesn't really matter if the Lord allowed it or caused it, we can still *"count it all joy when we encounter various trials"* (James 1:2).

So what benefits could possibly come through Jan's cancer? This book is intended to help us see these. Jan's faith was made stronger. My faith was made stronger. Our children's faith was made stronger. And many of you have said that your faith was made stronger. And without such faith, *"it is impossible to please God"* (Hebrews 11:6). Such faith is the basis of our rewards in eternity, which should be our desire anyway, and not a comfortable life on this hell-destined earth.

Cancer was Jan's megaphone to proclaim an uncommon faith. Whether God allowed it or caused it, cancer was Jan's platform to declare God's goodness despite outward circumstances, a message that would have had far less impact had cancer not been present.

Unfortunately, our faith often fails in the fiery furnace of adversity, because we choose not to believe in God's goodness, His trustworthiness, His eternal purposes. Perhaps we think of ourselves as good (though none are – Romans 3: 10-12) and undeserving of any hardship. Maybe we focus too much on earthly goals such as a comfortable house, a prosperous job, a secure retirement, or even a happy family.

But if we respond correctly, suffering can be our best classroom for learning character – endurance, patience, love, compassion, forgiveness, humility, obedience, contentment, loyalty, and many others. Because *"tribulation brings about perseverance, and perseverance, proven character"* (Romans 5:3-4), can't we, like Jan, welcome trials as our golden opportunity to make our testimony *"mature and complete, lacking in nothing"* (James 1:4)?

The hurts, struggles, and disappointments Jan encountered because of cancer at such a relatively young age are what magnified her character, highlighted her faith, and made her unwavering trust in God's goodness stand out. If the cancer had waited until she was a 70 year old retired missionary with no dependent children, it is doubtful her testimony would have been as powerful.

So did God merely allow Jan's cancer, or did He cause it? I don't know; Jan didn't know either. And it didn't matter to either of us, because our response would be the same either way. Whether Satan caused it and God allowed it (as happened in Job's case), or God planned it and caused it, we have complete trust in God's goodness to use it for our eternal benefit and His ultimate glory. The moment we enter heaven, with all its splendor and faith-earned rewards, we will be eternally grateful that God did it His way. *"Because Thy lovingkindness is better than life... so I will bless Thee as long as I live"* (Psalm 63:3-4).

Refined by Cancer

As you read Jan's October 3 update, look for clues that show Jan's awareness of God's benefits. And even when Jan doesn't see benefits, her faith still shines:

Greetings! I had an email prepared to go out last Saturday – and for your sake I wish it had (it would have been shorter).   But this past week has had 4 doctor visits, 1 MRI, and untold number of phone calls back and forth as ideas, questions, and discussion bounce around like a ball in a racquetball court.

The QUICK SUMMARY for those of you that have more to do than read my detailed medical saga – the "old" areas of cancer (liver, spleen, lungs, bones) are all still very small but stable / unchanged (with cancer gone in the kidney and uterus). A tumor in my gallbladder has increased significantly and is very active on the PET scan. MD Anderson Cancer Center doctors recommend surgery to remove the gallbladder as soon as possible. I see the surgeon on October 10; praying I can have surgery the 12th or 13th.

Another very active area is around the rod in my right hip. (Not surprising, as this is where my pain is.) MRI did not show any tumor but the rod makes the area difficult to see. We need to know definitively whether the pain / activity is due to swelling / inflammation or due to cancer in order to know what treatment to follow.

Now for those who want the details. What BLES-
SINGS I received last week when I went to MDAnderson
(the best cancer center in the U.S.) in Houston! Friends
(family in the Lord) provided a beautiful, restful place
to stay (with meals!), transported me back and forth
to the hospital and even went with me to consult the
oncologist (cancer specialist) on Friday.

Another friend stayed with me all day on Thursday
from 8 am to 5 pm (I was at the hospital from 6:45 am
to 7:45 pm). I had a PET scan, CT scans, blood work,
x-ray, and MRI. All the tests were done in a beautiful
new building where I had minimal walking. They even
had a nap room where I was able to sleep after lunch.
Believe it or not, I was even able to rest during the tests
(and pray!).

And of course, I visited with dear Filipino nurses
there, two of whom were from our area / of our dialect
group. Fun! I enjoyed really talking to them (in our
sweet sing-song language).

At the end of the day, one of the nurses escorted me
all the way to the ground lobby to wait for my friend.
Then I was able to visit Friday evening with 2 couples
that used to minister in the Philippines.

I am still researching and praying about another
systemic (for the whole body) treatment. MDAnderson
does not have any CLINICAL TRIALS at this time that
I qualify for; neither does the National Institutes of
Health, nor UCLA. The Lord knows whether I need any
more treatment or not.

When the FDA eliminated me from the trial, one
benefit that I could see through their decision is that it
allows people to see that God is in control of the healing.
That is why I chose Isaiah 42 in our last update -- *"I am
the LORD; that is my name! I will not give my glory
to another or my praise to idols."* Several people have
said that they feel that God has allowed this decision so
that He alone would receive glory and praise for what
He is doing in my life.

Now a family update. Thank you for praying for
MARTHA's birthday; she had a wonderful time with her
Sunday School class. Friends helped my girls decorate
with a "tropical" theme; refreshments were mini-hula

dancer spice cakes, fresh squeezed key lime juice, coconut ice cream balls, dried mangos, and fruit.

My dad and "second" mom Judy will visit us this week to celebrate SARA's 19th BIRTHDAY. The girls are planning a Victorian tea party with cucumber sandwiches and petit fours.

Hannah has experienced some discouragement recently. She says that she is feeling stressed and overwhelmed (guess who she takes after?). She sets high goals for herself.

Pray Philippines 4:8 for her -- that she would set her mind on what is true, right, pure, lovely, praiseworthy, etc. – and that she would recognize the lies of the enemy who seeks to destroy, kill, and steal her joy.

JONATHAN stays busy with Upward Soccer at our church, Tae Kwon Do, and pre-teen discipleship. He is also my partner for square dance lessons. Yes, despite the pain and limp, I told the children that I would take lessons if the Lord allowed me to be up and about, so I'm keeping my promise.

Jennifer Rothschild, in her Bible study Fingerprints of God, says that God uses affliction to mold, teach and nurture us. He allows these experiences "NOT TO DEFINE ME BUT TO REFINE ME." Yes! I don't want us to be known as the "missionary couple who both had cancer" but as God's children refined by cancer.

Psalm 66 says, *"Come and see what God has done, how awesome His works in man's behalf... He has preserved our lives and kept our feet from slipping. For you, O God, tested us: you refined us like silver... We went through fire and water, but you brought us to a place of abundance. Praise be to God, who has not rejected my prayer or withheld His love from me!"*

By October, 2006, we had been separated from our ministry and friends in the Philippines for more than a year. Although we maintained contact with several of our friends there, we longed to be back with them. You can clearly see Jan's heart for missions in her October 8 entry:

For you alert people who caught our typo in the last email, yes, I wrote PHILIPPINES instead of Philippians (when asking prayer for Hannah). I had two other proof readers -- but being family members, you can see where our mind is at! Now you can pray for the millions of Filipinos left without electricity or clean water because of typhoon Xangsane, which pummeled the Philippines last week. It was dubbed the cruelest typhoon since 1995, destroyed many homes and buildings and affected 53,685 people just around our city of Iloilo.

I wept last Sunday during our church service as we sang the song, *Send Us Out* -- as the church begins a month-long emphasis on missions. All I could think of was the many areas of the world in desperate spiritual darkness -- and here we are. I know that some people think we are crazy to even consider going back overseas, but God has not removed that missions call or desire from us.

We now have hanging in our living room a visual reminder of God's promise in Jeremiah 32:17. It is a beautiful Bierstadt print of the mountains to replace the one we left in the Philippines (purchased through the generous love gift of the oldest ladies' Sunday School class at Birchman Baptist). We affirm that: *"Ah, Sovereign LORD, you have made the heavens and the earth by your great power and outstretched arm. NOTHING IS TOO HARD FOR YOU."*

And I'm trusting that includes getting doctors to talk to each other about my care; I still don't have the hip biopsy arranged. Lord willing, I will have the gallbladder SURGERY AT BAYLOR University Medical Center in DALLAS, where I had my April surgery.

I was very pleased with the nursing staff there and already had a surgeon that I had consulted with earlier in the year. The surgery will probably need to be "open" due to the size of the tumor. So I'm preparing for that (longer recuperation period), but will be delightfully surprised if they can do laparoscopic surgery.

We so enjoyed our visit with DAD AND JUDY, although it was too short! They took the girls to the Hatshepsut Egyptian exhibit at the Kimbell Art Museum, accompanied me to a doctor visit, and watched Jonathan's Tae Kwon Do lesson. Judy fixed a great birthday supper for Sara. On their (LONG!) drive back to Virginia, they ate supper with David in Jackson, Tennessee and reported that he is doing fine (and busy!).

SARA also thoroughly enjoyed her lovely Victorian birthday tea party (planned and executed by Sara and her sisters and held at Peggy's sedate home). The girls made petit flour cakes, chocolate covered strawberries, tea cakes, chicken sandwiches and cucumber sandwiches, lemon ice with mint sprigs -- and, of course, also had English muffins and tea.

Friends of Peggy's let them borrow a lovely real silver tea set and antique porcelain tea cups. They and their guests dressed up in formals and Victorian dress -- even played in the park in their gowns! They had lots of fun!

So, where in the Bible is the Philippines? I suppose the reference is found in Isaiah 42:10 – *"Sing to the LORD a new song, His praise from the ends of the earth, you who go down to the sea, and all that is in it, you islands and all who live in them... Let them give glory to the LORD and proclaim His praise in the islands."*

May Psalm 97 be our prayer this week: *"The LORD reigns; let the earth rejoice; Let the many islands be glad... Light is sown like seed for the righteous, and gladness for the upright in heart. Be glad in the LORD, you righteous ones; and give thanks to His holy name."*

Jan had her gallbladder removed on Friday, the 13th (we were not superstitious). Sara provided the next Caringbridge update on the 15th:

Hiya everyone! Wow, it's been a long time since I last wrote an update! Time has passed so quickly lately, and I, for one, cannot believe that we have been here in the States for 16 months! I cannot also believe that I am now a college student and newly turned 19 years old; I feel so old...

College is going great for me; I'm enjoying my classes (four design classes...15 hours!) and have made several new friends. I would ask for prayer though, for my classmates; because as of right now, I do not believe any of them are Christians and I see some of them living lives that are ungodly; I feel burdened for them. I am trying to be the best influence I can right now, and hopefully I'll be able to find the right moment to talk with them about God.

Mom's surgery went very well! They were able to do it laparoscopically (not sure of my spelling here) and the surgeons successfully removed her gallbladder. The gallbladder contained 3 marble sized tumors. It is an AMAZING blessing that the tumors had not caused any problems or blockages in the gallbladder (besides of course, being cancerous!).

Mom is now at Aunt Peggy's lovely home (we love you Aunt Peggy!!!) and enjoying a little R&R, music, and the Bible. She slept 12 hours the first night; a feat that has not been accomplished in quite awhile! Mom's Uncle Mike was down from Oregon for awhile and he brought Chinese take-out for supper on Saturday at Aunt Peggy's... you'll be pleased to note that we kids were in attendance, too!

Wedgwood has been having a mission focused month (as mentioned in a previous update, if I am correct) and this past Sunday night featured the flags from Spain, Ecuador, and the Philippines. We were emailed about holding the flags and so Martha held the Ecuadorian flag, Jonathan the Spanish flag, and I had the Philippine flag (it was a hotly debated subject in our family as to who would get the Philippine flag... I got it since I was oldest).

On Tuesday Mom will go and see the oncologist and try to determine what the next course of action should be, like therapy. Friday, Mom will go and talk to the WMU at Connell Baptist Church. Please pray she'll be feeling good that day!

I usually sit in the hall before and in between my classes (as all my classes are in one hall). As I was sitting there one day, reading, a classmate walked by on his way to another class...he jokingly asked if I had a home, since I am always sitting in the same spot. I replied that of course I did...but then when he was gone,

I was left to reflect on his question and my response.

I don't have a real earthly home at the moment; (the kind of home that my classmate was referring to), but I do have a heavenly home, and that knowledge has given me comfort. My family doesn't know where we will be living a year from now, but we know that wherever we are, we have a secure home in heaven waiting for us; and while we are here on earth, God will always be taking care of us.

We so very much covet and appreciate your prayers! You don't know how much you have been a blessing to our family (even those of you that we have never met in person). The biggest way you can help us is by praying!! Thank you so much for supporting us, we love you all so much!

God Will Make a Way

Christian faith is not the absence of doubt or discouragement. Rather, it is a steadfast trust in the Lord, Jesus Christ, especially when doubt and discouragement tempt us to question His goodness. Follow Jan in her October 28, 2006, entry as she turns her discouragement into a Biblically based testimony of faith:

God is serious about not giving another His glory or His praise to idols (anything that takes the place of God in our lives). I still don't have a treatment plan in place – it has now been over 4 months since my last cancer vaccine and 1½ months since I would have received my last vaccine.

Since the last update, I found out about a monoclonal antibody clinical trial (the new "wave" of treatment for melanoma) in Dallas that my local oncologist, MD Anderson oncologists, and the prior clinical trial doctor all felt would be good for me since it targets the immune system.

I interviewed with the new trial, but when the doctors discussed my case, they felt that it would not be suitable for me. So I am still seeking, still praying, still asking.

It has been a stressful 2 weeks. The orthopedic oncologist finally talked to the MDAnderson oncologist about the hip biopsy – 3 days AFTER my gallbladder surgery. He was willing to work me in for surgery last week, but my surgeon didn't think that I needed to have another surgery so soon, especially since it would be an open incision and not needle biopsy. (More possibilities of problems.) So that biopsy is on hold. But praise God that the hip is feeling better; I think because I have seen a lymph drainage therapist. It seems that the pain is related to swelling – a side effect of the radiation and surgery.

Never have I felt so desperately in need of God's direction. Yes, it has been discouraging; I have felt tempted to just give up the effort to search for treatment. At the same time, I know that God is in control and in His timing, He will show me the right thing to do.

I talk to people who get our updates and they think that I never get down. No, I have my moments. But I go back again to God's Word which is TRUTH – not the discouraging lies of the enemy, not the dismal statistics of the cancer doctors, not just "thinking positive thoughts" philosophy. God's Word gets me focused again on Jesus, the author and perfecter of our faith. His promises reassure me, comfort me, challenge me, calm me.

Let me show you how God did that this past week. I woke Tuesday with the song *God Will Make a Way* going through my head. Maybe this is how Zephaniah 3:17 is true in my life – *"The Lord your God is with you, He is mighty to save. He will take great delight in you, He will quiet you with His love, He will rejoice over you with singing."*

Often the praise songs that we sing are based on Scripture (it is His word, so God does sing to us through them). Using this song, I looked up Scripture references to it. I knew that Isaiah 43 had references to roads in the wilderness so I started there.

As I read through the Word, I dialogued (sometimes with tears) with God over it – asking and answering questions. God says, *"Forget the former things; do not dwell on the past.* (Past treatment?) *See I am doing a new thing! Now it springs up; do you not perceive it?"* (Is. 43: 19).   I responded, *"No, Lord, I don't see yet what you are doing or what direction I am to take."* God continues, *"I am making a way in the desert and streams in the wasteland (for what purpose, God?)... to give drink to my people, my chosen, the people I formed for myself that they may proclaim my praise"* (Is. 43:20-21).

God reminded me anew of His purpose for me in this cancer journey – to proclaim His praise, to show forth His glory. Here are the other Scriptures that comforted me and set my feet firmly back on the Rock:

God will make a way, where there seems to be no way.
He works in ways we cannot see;
He will make a way for me.

> *"My ways are not your ways, declares the Lord. I will tell you of new things, of hidden things unknown to you. No eye has seen, no mind has conceived what God has prepared for those who love Him"* (Isaiah 55:8; Isaiah 48:6; 1 Cor. 2:9).

He will be my guide; hold me closely to His side.
With love and strength for each new day,
He will make a way. God will make a way.

> *"He will be my guide even to the end. The Lord stood at my side and gave me strength. O LORD, we long for you. Be our strength every morning. In all their distress, He too was distressed... In His love and mercy He redeemed them; He lifted them up and carried them all the days of old. It is God who arms me with strength and makes my way perfect"* (Psalm 48:14; 2 Timothy 4:17; Isaiah 33:2; Isaiah 63:9; Psalm 18:32).

By a roadway in the wilderness He leads me.
And rivers in the desert will I see.
Heaven and earth will fade.
But His Word will still remain.
And He will do something new today.

> *"Some wandered in desert wastelands...The LORD led them by a straight way. I will make rivers flow on barren heights... so that people may see and know that the hand of the LORD has done this. In the beginning you laid the foundations of the earth, and the heavens are the work of your hand. They will perish, but you will remain. The Word of our God stands forever."* (Psalm 107:4; Isaiah 41:18, 20; Psalm 102:25; Isaiah 40:8)

God will make a way, where there seems to be no way.
He works in ways we cannot see;
He will make a way for me.

> *"The highway in the wilderness will be called the way of Holiness... the redeemed will enter Zion with singing; ...gladness and joy will overtake them, and sorrow and sighing will flee away. Whether you turn to the right or to the left, you will hear a voice behind you, saying, 'This is the way; walk in it.'"* (Isaiah 35: 8-10; Isaiah 30:21)

He will be my guide, hold me closely to His side.
With love and strength for each new day,
He will make a way. God will make a way.

The Secret to Jan's Faith

Posted on our bathroom door (a place where family members pass by at least three times a day), is a list of gifts we have received in the past two years. Jan called it our Psalm 37:25 fund: *"...I have never seen the righteous forsaken or their children begging for bread."*

Posted are about 130 tangible reminders of God's watch-care over us. Some are just a few dollars. A few are over a thousand dollars. But each one has been a faith builder for our family and a continual reminder that God's faithfulness knows no end.

Added to this is the list written in heaven of all the loving people who have brought us food, taken the kids out shopping, given us clothes, cared for our children, and most importantly – prayed for us regularly. Each one of these expressions of love has been a building block in our testimony of God's faithfulness. We were a family truly blessed.

Once again, blessings and faith are Jan's theme in her November 28, 2006, update:

Happy Thanksgiving! May God open our spiritual eyes to see His blessings, not just in material or physical areas. *"Praise be to the God and Father of our Lord Jesus Christ, who has blessed us in the heavenly realms with EVERY spiritual blessing in Christ"*. Here are just a few of the blessings that Paul lists in Ephesians 1:

> *In love He predestined us to be adopted as His sons...*
> *He has freely given us His glorious grace...*
> *In Him we have redemption...the forgiveness of sins...*
> *He made known to us the mystery of His will.*
> *In Him we were also chosen, having been predestined according to the plan of Him who works out everything in conformity with the purpose of His will, in order that we might be for the praise of His glory...*

See how we keep coming back to God's purpose of bringing Him glory in our lives?

Last May, I was asked by a reporter, *"Have there been UNEXPECTED BLESSINGS in walking a path that no one would choose?"*

One of the unexpected incredible blessings has been the PEOPLE who have poured out their love on us. We never knew that we had so many friends willing to sacrifice for us. Not only our friends, but people and churches that we have never met face to face.

When this all started in 2004, Martha (then 11 years old) asked, *"Why are people so nice to us?"* I still don't really understand, but I believe that one way that God has shown His presence to us is when His people minister to our family in His name.

"Lord, when did we see you hungry... or thirsty... or a stranger... or needing clothes... or sick? The King will reply, "I tell you the truth, whatever you did for one of the least of these brothers of mine, you did for me" (Matt 25: 37-40).

Thank you for being His hands, His heart, His feet as you have ministered to us, one of the least – and so undeserving of His mercies.

We are studying the book of Hebrews at our church's Sunday morning Bible study. Hebrews 11 and 12 have been central to my walk of faith through this cancer 'journey.' After the enemy spent a few days trying to shake me up, how refreshing it was to be "in the Lord's house" and reminded of the TRUTH in Hebrews 11: *"Faith is being SURE of what we hope for and CERTAIN of what we do not see."* In fact, I cried all through the reading of Hebrews 11 as God reminded me again of His perspective.

What am I sure of? I am SURE that God is in control; He sits on His throne and does what pleases Him. He is Sovereign and He knows the plans that He has for me. I am SURE that God acts according to His character, which is loving, faithful, trustworthy, holy, merciful, righteous, all-knowing, all-powerful.

It is proper on a day like today, to reflect on what God has done for us – that keeps me going! Last Thanksgiving, we made our own family version of Psalm 136, where we listed characteristics of God and what He has done for us. Try it -- and keep it as a reminder of God's faithfulness and that God is at work in your life.

I may not always see HOW God is working, but I am CERTAIN that He is. Those in the "roll call of faithful" in Hebrews 11 *"were all commended for their faith, yet none of them received what had been promised. God had planned something better for us so that only together with us would they be made perfect."*

This is a mystery yet to me, but God has planned something BETTER for us – and it somehow involves them, you, others who have ministered to us, and me as we *"run with perseverance the race set before us."* None of us are in this alone. God is doing something that involves all of you that He has brought forth to support us in prayer.

But most importantly, there is Jesus, *"the author and perfecter of our faith, who for the JOY set before Him endured the cross"*. As you have heard me say before, "Let us FIX OUR EYES on Jesus" – this is what helps me get my perspective back when Satan tries to rattle and shake me. How can you pray for me? That I keep my eyes fixed on Jesus – when treatment are uncertain, when the pain intensifies in my hip, when the children struggle with insecurity about our future, etc.

I am finishing up 2 weeks of self-injections of a drug currently in clinical trials to prevent the growth of melanoma cancer (the mission board doctor worked with insurance and our benefits department to get it approved – praise God!). I can now be thankful for all that excess skin around my middle from having such big babies – it makes a great pin cushion.

David is home for a few days before heading back to the end of the semester busyness. Lord willing, we will go to my dad's house in Virginia for Christmas. (And a doctor last year said that Christmas 2005 would be my last. Doctors don't have the last word – God does!)

"I sought the LORD, and He answered me; He delivered me from all my fears. Those who look to Him are radiant; their faces are never covered with shame" (Ps. 34:4-5).

Pain in Jan's right leg increased during November. An x-ray on December 1 showed a new fracture. This indicated the cancer was growing. From this point on, Jan had to use a walker, or be pushed in a wheelchair. Perhaps Jan sensed her time was near. Ignoring the destruction in her leg, she made plans to travel to Virginia for Christmas, including a week long vacation just for our family at a private Christian camp in Kentucky.

What was the secret to Jan's faith? It should be obvious that one cannot maintain a strong faith apart from regular meditation in God's Word. Passages such as Psalm 1 and Joshua 1:8 explain that daily communion with God through His Word is the only way to maintain an enduring faith. On December 2, the day after she learned of her new fracture, Jan shares her meditation and application of Psalm 31...

(verse 10) *"My strength fails because of my affliction, and my bones grow weak."*

Due to increasing pain in my right leg, I went to the ER yesterday for an x-ray. There is a new fracture line which "appears to be" continued destruction of the bone (like a fracture due to osteoporosis / thinning bone).

The good news is that with my "impressive hardware" (that big rod in my thigh that runs from top of the hip to my knee), the leg can't just break, so the fracture is considered stable. I can't put any weight on that leg, but I can shuffle pretty well with my walker. Pray that my right elbow (which also has a small area of bone destruction) will stay strong enough to bear the weight. More good news - the children think it's neat that we have a handicap parking sticker.

(verse 14) *"But I trust in you, O LORD; I say, "You are MY God."*

Do you get it? We serve a very personal God. He knows me intimately and cares about me. (And you too!) On disappointing days, I choose to REMEMBER who God is and what He has done for me. He is MY strength, MY rock, MY fortress, MY deliverer, MY shield, MY salvation, MY stronghold, MY refuge, MY hope, MY honor, MY help, MY confidence (Psalm 18, 28, 31, 62, 63, 71 – and there are more!).

Don't you love that word "confidence"? *"So we say with confidence, 'the Lord is my helper; I will not be afraid. What can man do to me?'"* (Hebrews 13:6). Martha quoted this verse in a skit the youth did last Sunday night. Pray that her total trust will be in God regarding the future.

(verse 15) *"My times are in your hands..."*

He KNOWS my times! He knows that on my schedule this week are repeat PET / CT scans and MRI to determine if the cancer is growing, stable or shrinking. He knows the results already. If growing, then I will need to travel for another clinical trial, but

I'll wait until after our Christmas trip to Virginia. Pray that even now He is working out those details in HIS perfect timing (Ecclesiastes 3).

(verse 16) *"Let your face shine on your servant; save me in your unfailing love."*
Even in the ER and in pain, He is with me. Pray that as His face shines on me, I will reflect His glory. *"We, who with unveiled faces all reflect the Lord's glory, are being transformed into His likeness with ever-increasing glory, which comes from the Lord"* (2 Corinthians 3:18).

(verse 17) *"Let me not be put to shame, O LORD, for I have cried out to you."*
"I eagerly expect and hope that I will in no way be ashamed, but will have sufficient courage so that now as always Christ will be exalted in my body" (Phil. 1:20).

(verse 19) *"How great is your goodness, which you have stored up for those who fear you."*
How good God is! Sara was nominated and received an award from her college (Tarrant County Community College) for "Distinguished Student Scholar." It should provide enough for her books / computer programs for the next semester. What an honor and affirmation of her diligence and talent. My unmotivated student – who never wanted to go to college – confessed that she likes college and is really enjoying her studies in computer graphic design. How great God is!

(verse 24) *"Be strong and take heart, all you who HOPE in the LORD."*
Tomorrow morning, we will be sharing at South Park Baptist in Grand Prairie. I suppose I have an excuse to stay home (a leg fracture), but I don't want to miss an opportunity to share of the HOPE that is within me. Pray that the Holy Spirit would prepare the hearts of those who will come and He will give us just the right words to say. *"May the God of hope fill you with all joy and peace as you trust in Him, so that you may overflow with hope by the power of the Holy Spirit"* (Romans 15:13).

I would love to hear from you. I have about 4 hours of scan time this week where I need to lay still. Let me know how I can pray for you.

Did you catch those last couple of sentences? Read them again. For an MRI scan, Jan had to lay still on a small, moveable, flatbed. With arms by her side, the flatbed slid her inside what I describe as a giant PVC pipe, a hollow tube with absolutely nothing to look at except colorless curved plastic four inches from your nose. The loud kackling noise of the MRI machine left no chance for sleep.

Jan's routine was to keep her eyes closed the entire time, and pray, not just for herself, but for her family, for her friends, for you. I know this because on the way home, she would share with me some of the things she prayed for and the insights the Lord gave her while she prayed.

Humor

By now you know that Jan could find humor in just about anything. We often joked about the possibility of Jan getting high on her morphine pain medication. However, because she was careful with the dosage, she never had any side effects, until now.

It was a Thursday evening. Jan had a dinner date with a lady from her Bible study group. But the pastor had requested a drop-by visit with our family that evening to check on how we were doing. Jan figured she could be done with dinner and back home in time for the pastor's visit.

As dinner was served (she had to take morphine with food) Jan made a quick calculation that she had just enough morphine left in the medicine bottle for one dosage. Without measuring it, she just gulped the remaining medication directly from the bottle, thinking that it sure felt like more than one dosage. It was.

By the time Jan came home, she was happy! Moments later, the pastor arrived. Jan was as giddy as ever. She talked and laughed, which was not unusual for Jan, but I could tell a difference. Jan was feeling good!

The pastor stayed for about twenty minutes with Jan dominating the conversation. However, moments before he left, Jan became unusually quiet. As soon as the front door shut, Jan turned a different color, hobbled quickly to the bathroom, and lost her dinner.

Far from being embarrassed, Jan later thought the whole incident made a hilarious story. She even told it to her oncologist, the one who had prescribed the morphine.

Jan's December 10, 2006, entry is another example of her great sense of humor:

Scientists now know that laughter boosts your immune system – proving what was written in Proverbs 17:22 many thousands of years ago. While we are waiting for my scan results, I thought the following story might bring a smile. Try and visualize it for a good laugh.

Banging and thumping of the bedroom wall startled me awake. I was recuperating from my gallbladder surgery at Peggy's house. It sounded like Peggy was opening the drawers of her dresser and slamming them shut. What had happened to her? The wall was practically vibrating; I pressed my ear to it and listened intently, but couldn't figure out the sounds.

Finally I decided to check on her. Cautiously, I opened the door but couldn't see if Peggy was in her bed. Knowing that Peggy kept a shotgun under her bed (a remnant of her ranch days), I flipped the light on, then heard something in the hallway.

I whipped my head around and Peggy was stealthily stalking down the hallway, not with her shotgun but with a broom in hand. She had also been wakened by the noises; she thought it sounded like someone walking on the roof.

We stood there, mouths open, with our faces lifted up to the ceiling, straining to discern. When we would talk, the thumping would stop. When we were quiet, we could hear the movement across the roof again. We whispered our theories and concerns. Peggy had had some workmen out to repair her roof; wild thoughts were running through her head that they were trying to get in the house, thinking she was alone.

Peggy suggested we call 9-11. *"Should we change our clothes?"* I asked. *"No,"* she said, *"I've done this before. We only need to brush our teeth."* So she rushed off to rinse her mouth with Listerine, while I quickly brushed my teeth.

Soon the police car arrived. The officer slowly drove around the house, scanning the roof with his spotlight. Peggy went out to meet him while I stood in the doorway.

He explained that there were 3 big fat raccoons on the roof. They had torn all the wood shingles off in two places—one over Peggy's bed and one over my bed. Peggy started to explain to the officer in detail, as only Peggy can do, about her house, her roofing problems, and the workmen, but I thanked the officer for coming and he left.

When Peggy came back in the house, she realized that we were both wearing look-alike "old lady" robes. Her robe had belonged to her mother (and Peggy is 78 years old) and mine had belonged to my grandmother (who would be 92 years old if she was still living). We began to laugh at how silly we must have looked to the police officer – and what he thought about these two matching ladies so frightened by raccoons.

We decided that to capture the moment, we had to have our picture made. So – ta-dah! Here is our picture, [at the beginning of this chapter] compliments of Wal-Mart's $5.98 special. The pictures almost didn't get made; the photographer had to take a break when we were laughing so hard telling our story that my face got red.

Now we have a reminder of how much fun we can have just being silly (although when the wall rattled, it seemed quite serious).

I hope when you look at your problems today that you too can find humor in your situation. Remember: Today is a gift – that's why it is called THE PRESENT!"

Family Times

Despite the growing pain in her right leg, Jan was determined to enjoy our family vacation. Knowing we would be gone for more than two weeks, Jan filled our final week in Fort Worth with a slate of doctor visits.

One visit was to the doctor who had developed the dendritic cell vaccine. He assured Jan that, although she was out of the clinical trial, the vaccine was still working. She should not consider any other systemic treatment at this time, because it might interfere with the vaccine.

On Thursday, December 14, 2006, in what would be her last journal entry, Jan shared our travel plans and the results of her latest scans:

We are so thankful for our Southern Baptist supporters. This month Southern Baptist Churches collect a special offering (called the Lottie Moon Christmas Offering) for international missions. Our 5000+ missionaries depend on these funds each year for their salary, housing, vehicles, evangelistic projects, and medical needs (like us!!!).

We are seeing amazing growth among people groups that were unreached in years past. Just a few dollars can go a long way in providing basic support and resources for those who serve in difficult places.

Speaking of giving, since coming to the U.S., we have been on the receiving end of so many gifts, and this Christmas season is no exception. In the past two weeks, we have received three large gifts that will be enough for a few months of our nutraceutical supplements (that's helping to keep us relatively healthy) and to give each child some nice Christmas gifts. Thank you, you angels in disguise. We take these gifts as reminders of God's goodness to us and of His continual presence.

We sure will appreciate your prayers as we travel to Kentucky and Virginia. This Friday, the girls and I will fly to Tennessee, where some friends will drive us to Cleft Rock Retreat Center in Kentucky. Pray that I can be a blessing to those who wheelchair me around and assist me.

Saturday, Mark and Jonathan will drive to Jackson, TN, where they will meet up with David and then join us Sunday in Kentucky. Pray that we will have quality family time, talking about the past year and praying about the future.

Then Thursday, Dec. 21, we will drive to a church camp in Virginia, where we will join my dad and step-mom, her two sons and her daughter-in-law, my younger brother and his wife. My older brother Wynn will also be driving in from Texas with his wife and two daughters. My step-mom has decorated the camp, planned family activities and food -- now the only thing else we would like is some snow!

December 27, we will be visiting Buffalo Junction Baptist Church -- one of the many Southern Baptist Churches that has been so supportive of our family. Mark and the boys will then head back to Texas; the girls and I will stay in Virginia until January 1.

Now, for my scan reports. Overall, things look really good! No tumors visible in any organ now except for the spleen and those in the spleen are still small and stable (haven't grown since March). My brain is still "unremarkable" -- that translates as no cancer there and again, an amazing blessing! So I still have no "measurable disease" that would qualify me for a clinical trial.

However, the right hip still shows much activity on the PET scan, correlating with continued destruction of the right thigh bone as well as soft tissue. We saw the orthopedic oncologist on Monday and an x-ray shows even more destruction of the bone from the December 1 x-ray. My former clinical trial oncologist and my radiologist both recommend a hip and femur (thigh bone) replacement. So pray with us about the decision to do another surgery in January.

For the next two weeks, I'm going to try and put all these decisions out of my mind. I'm going to enjoy my family, food, and fun (as much as my "bum" leg will let me). No skiing or basketball! I'm going to remember that *"unto us a child is born, unto us a Son is given...and*

His Name IS Wonderful Counselor, Mighty God, Eternal Father, Prince of Peace" (Is. 9:6).

This speaks to me of the wisdom that He will give us in decision making, His power to use all things for good in our lives to conform us to the image of Jesus Christ, of our "Abba" Father who has loved me with an everlasting love, and of the peace that Jesus gives us for our journey everyday.

The next day, I took Jan and the girls to the airport for their flight to Tennessee, where friends would drive them to the Christian camp. From a distance, I watched Jan make her way through airport security in her wheelchair. The agent slowly moved his metal detector over Jan's arms and legs, obviously concerned about his readings. Jan was quite animated as she described her "impressive metal hardware". After about five minutes, the agent released her, convinced that this handicapped lady with three teenage girls was no terrorist.

The following day, Jonathan and I drove to Tennessee and spent the night with David in his dorm room. After worship on Sunday, we drove to Kentucky, meeting up with the rest of our family that night. For four days and nights, we stayed in a newly built home (owned by missionaries). The camp was quiet, the food was great, and the camp owners were marvelous. In addition to our leisure activities, we had quality family times as we discussed our feelings and what we had learned from the past year and a half of our cancer adventure.

On Thursday, the 21st, we toured the Cumberland Gap area as we made our way to the church camp twenty minutes south of Jan's hometown of Vinton, Virginia. Our time with Jan's side of the family was relaxed. Again, the food was great, as family members pitched in to help Judy prepare. We watched movies, played games, and told stories. On Sunday, we attended worship at Bill and Judy's church, then opened gifts the following morning on Christmas Day.

On Wednesday, Jan, the girls, and I drove to Buffalo Junction Baptist Church, near the border of North Carolina, where several members had kept up with us over the years. After another delicious meal, Jan and I had the opportunity to briefly share about missions and about our cancer adventure. We had a great time of fellowship.

Early the next morning, David, Jonathan, and I packed the car in preparation for our long drive back to Fort Worth. We wanted to buy David a used car in Fort Worth on Saturday, the last day of the month and of the year (great deals!). Jan and the girls would be flying back to Fort Worth on Monday, the 1st, so we would only be separated for a few days. We gave Jan hugs as we double checked the luggage. With Jan standing outside in the cold morning wind, smiling, holding on to her walker, we waved goodbye.

Later that day, Jan, Sara, Hannah, and Martha, along with Bill and Judy, left the church camp and drove back to Vinton, to the house where Jan had been raised. Because of her leg, Jan slept in the downstairs bedroom, while the girls slept upstairs in a bedroom next to Bill and Judy's.

On Sunday, Jan and the girls worshiped at Vinton Baptist Church. Sunday was a special day because it was Jan's 50th birthday. They celebrated in the evening with a festive family meal at Red Lobster Inn. Wearing a birthday hat, Jan was her jovial self, even getting into a food slinging spar with those sitting across from her. Laughs were shared as well as stories. It was a fabulous birthday celebration.

Back at the house, Jan packed. They would leave for the airport at 7 a.m. At midnight, as fireworks were going off around the city, Hannah and Martha relaxed in the den with Mom. For over an hour they talked about the Philippines, about school, about the future. Martha went up to bed. Moments later, Hannah hugged Mom good night and went upstairs to bed as Mom, using her walker, made her way to her downstairs bedroom. It was 1:30 a.m., and Jan was an hour and a half into her year of Jubilee.

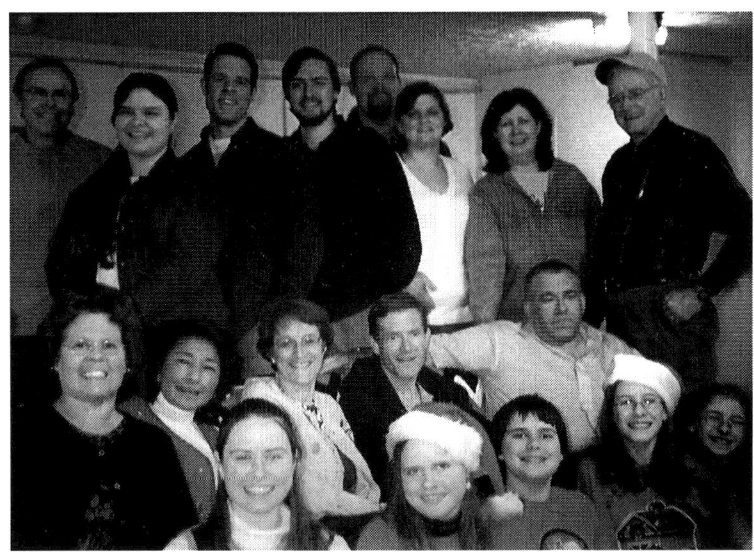

Jan's family - Christmas Eve 2006

Chapter 10: "I'VE BEEN READY FOR A LONG TIME"

It was 3:15 a.m. Judy heard the knocking first. *"Bill, there's someone at the door."*

From their second floor bedroom window, Bill looked outside. An ambulance and a police car ware parked outside the house, flashing their multicolored lights.

"It must be Jan," Bill thought. They hurried down the stairs to the front door, passing the opened door to Jan's bedroom. She wasn't there.

Judy opened the door for the paramedics who said that they had received a 911 call from this residence.

They found Jan on the other side of the house, in the den, collapsed on the floor, just under the telephone. She had vomited several times.

While the paramedics went to work, Judy rushed up the stairs to get the girls. She came to Hannah first. *"Get dressed! Your mother is going to the emergency room!"*

Hannah came down the stairs in time to see the paramedics lifting Jan onto the stretcher. Jan's eyes were closed, but she kept mumbling, *"White bag; red folder. White bag; red folder."* Hannah knew that to be Mom's medical records. She grabbed the bag. Bill and Hannah got into the car and followed the ambulance to the hospital.

Jan later explained that shortly after Hannah went upstairs to bed, her head began hurting. She tried for nearly an hour to sleep, but couldn't. As her head pain increased she became nauseated. When she got out of bed the pain increased even more. She couldn't climb the stairs because of her leg, so she called out for help. But everyone was asleep; no one could hear her.

Jan was making her way toward the bathroom, just off the den, when her food came up. The pressure of vomiting caused excruciating pain in her head. She fell on the den floor, then crawled her way to the telephone. She had to call 911 twice before she could mumble out the words of her address. Then the ambulance came.

January 1 is one of the busiest days for any hospital. The New Year's Eve celebrations are over. The hospital emergency room is filled with victims of defective fireworks, automobile accidents, and drunken parties.

The sun was coming up when nurses and doctors finally gave Jan their attention. A head CT scan was quickly ordered. Judy had arrived with Sara and Martha. At 7:30 a.m., the doctor told Bill that, according to the scan results, Jan had a large pool of blood inside the lower back portion of her head. She had suffered a brain hemorrhage. Immediate surgery would be necessary to stop further bleeding. A neurosurgeon had been summoned.

Brain Surgery

Back in Fort Worth, Judy had called me shortly after the ambulance left for the emergency room. I was hoping it was just a complication with her medications. But Hannah's call at 7:30 told me otherwise. Two hours later, before the surgery, I spoke briefly over the telephone with the surgeon. I then sent out a mass email to everyone on our prayer list:

It's Monday morning, 11 a.m. [10 a.m. central time]. David, Jonathan, and I drove back to Ft. Worth from Virginia on Friday, after a wonderful Christmas time with family. Jan and the girls are still in Virginia and were scheduled to fly back to Ft. Worth this afternoon.

Shortly after midnight, Jan began experiencing head pain and nausea. She could not climb the stairs of her father's house, so she was unable to alert her family upstairs. She called 911. The ambulance and police woke Jan's father and step-mother. They found her collapsed on the floor in the den, barely able to speak (but Jan still had the presence of mind to explain where her medical records were). I was called at around 4:30 a.m and told that Jan was in the emergency room, with Jan's father and Hannah nearby. We were hoping that it was just some complications from her medications.

At 7:30, Hannah called and said the CT scan showed a blood pool in the lower back portion of the brain, and that a neurosurgeon was on his way. About 30 minutes ago, I talked to the neurosurgeon who confirmed that Jan had experienced some hemorrhaging near the brain stem, near the portion of the brain that controlled coordination and balance, not the portion that controlled thinking processes. A blood clot had formed, but there was a high risk that the hemorrhaged area may be pressing on the stem and impeding or blocking the flow of cerebral fluids.

So, Jan will be having surgery later this morning to remove the hemorrhaged fluids and hopefully repair the weakened blood vessels. The doctor said that while this is not technically a stroke, it acts somewhat like a stroke. The extent of any brain damage from the hemorrhage will not be fully known for several days. Recovery may take weeks to months.

Please pray now for the surgeon. Pray that Jan comes through the surgery fine and with full thinking capabilities. We will start packing and leave for Virginia this afternoon, after we hear the results of the surgery. I will post the results on www.caringbridge.com/tx/moses.

Of course, I am very concerned for Jan right now; lots of thoughts racing through my mind. But as the

Lord so faithfully does, He gives grace when we need it most. And right now, I know the Lord is with Jan and with each of us, gently and lovingly walking with us each step of the way.

In Virginia, a large group of family and friends filled the surgical waiting room. In Texas, the boys and I were quickly packing. Two hours later, the surgery was over and I posted the following Caringbridge entry:

As I mentioned on the previous update, Jan was taken to the emergency room in Roanoke, Virginia, hours before she and the girls were scheduled to fly back to Ft. Worth, where David, Jonathan, and I arrived on Friday.

The neurosurgeon said that Jan's hemorrhage was rather large, but the blood clot was removed and that, for now, she was OK. She will remain in ICU. for the next two to three days to watch for any further hemorrhaging. The doctor had no explanation for the hemorrhaging, saying it may or may not be cancer related.

As I mentioned previously, the neurosurgeon said that this kind of brain hemorrhaging often acts like a stroke, so we will not know the extent of any damage until a few days into her recovery.

Sara, Hannah, and Martha said they were doing fine, enjoying pizza for lunch. David, Jonathan, and I will leave this afternoon to return to Virginia.

I will plan to write an update sometime Wednesday.

When Jan's cancer returned in May of 2004, one of her first prayer requests was that she would make it to her 50th birthday, her Year of Jubilee (God's Old Testament designation for every 50th year to be the year for freedom). That prayer was answered on Sunday, her 50th birthday.

Another one of her prayer requests was that she would retain her ability to think and speak clearly regardless of what happened with the rest of her body. Please be in prayer for this request.

We don't have a crystal ball to know what will happen next. But because of our faith in Jesus, one is not needed. God is not surprised by this. We know Jan is firmly in the Lord's hands – no better place to be.

Jan was taken to the recovery room where she was given medication to keep her sedated through the night. She was placed on a ventilator and had a feeding tube inserted through her nose down to her stomach. Judy and Sara stayed with her for about an hour, but Jan was still in a drug induced sleep. That night everyone slept.

While they were sleeping, David and I took turns driving through the night. We arrived in Roanoke the following morning at 10:30 a.m. Judy directed us to the hospital where Bill and the girls were waiting with Jan. What I remember most was Jan's coughing. Fluid had built up in her lungs but she lacked the muscle strength to cough it up. A nurse had to insert a plastic tube down her throat to suction the fluids. The coughing caused severe pain in Jan's head.

Jan could open her eyes, but they would roll back and forth, unable to focus. She could point with her fingers, but was unable to lift up her arm. Obviously, the hemorrhage had caused extensive short term damage. Long term damage could not yet be determined. We were all wondering if the hemorrhage had affected her thinking.

She kept pointing to her white bag. One by one, we lifted items from her bag. Jan, with barely perceptible movements of her head, kept responding *no*. We emptied her bag without any positive response from Jan. Finally, when someone mentioned "plane tickets", she nodded *yes*. Jan was concerned about their missed flight. Well, at least her memory seemed fine.

That evening, January 2, 2007, I added to our journal:

I just returned from the ICU of Roanoke Memorial Hospital. Jan's condition is listed as serious but stable. It is not a stroke or aneurysm. Neither does it seem to be cancer related. The doctor's best guess at this point is that the hemorrhaging was due to AVM - Arterio-Venous Malformation, a congenital tangle of abnormal and poorly formed blood vessels that weaken with age. At some point, as in Jan's case, they can rupture and damage brain tissue.

While the surgery removed most of the pooled blood, it will take another 4 to 6 weeks for Jan's body to absorb the remaining cerebral fluids. Only then will we know the full extent of brain damage. The doctor was encouraged this afternoon that Jan could respond to simple commands, such as moving, to some degree, her arms, hands, and legs. Her breathing is labored, she has bouts of intense pain, but she can open her eyes and make attempts to communicate.

At this point, we are looking at maybe several weeks in the hospital, followed by rehabilitation, then home care. Of course, the cancer issues remain - her right leg lesions, possible hip replacement, follow-up scans, and some form of systemic treatment. A lot to deal with.

But this evening, I brought Jan's audio CD's and a player to the hospital. She was able to point to the CD she wanted to listen to, a CD of 100 Promises from God's Word.

I am confident that Jan's faith will remain strong. Mine, too. But emotions have a way of making truth a bit foggy at times, and it is so hard for me to see Jan suffer like this. And I know it is even more difficult for Jan not to be able to communicate, the one ability she so earnestly prayed would stay intact.

All the children are here with me. School starts next week. Lots of decisions to make. I will purpose to post another update tomorrow evening.

Cautious Optimism

Initially, we did not think the hemorrhage was cancer related. Her December MRI brain scanned detected no cancer activity.

By the third day, her breathing seemed to stabilize somewhat and we could see small improvements in her arm coordination. The surgeon felt confident that, if her breathing remained stable, she could be air transported to Fort Worth in a few days. Still, he cautioned that recovery would take months, if not longer. I was still wondering about her mental abilities.

Jan started pointing to her white bag again. I took out her wallet. She nodded *yes*.

I asked, *"Is it one of your calling cards?"*

Another nod *yes*.

I flipped through her dozens of cards, naming each one and waiting for Jan's response. She lifted her finger when I read her Restless Leg Syndrome (RLS) Medical Alert Card.

Then I remembered. Yesterday, one of the nurses mentioned *Phenergan* as the medication she was placing in Jan's I.V. to control her nausea. Jan had tried to communicate something.

"Is it the Phenergan?" I asked. Jan smiled and gave a thumbs up. Her RLS Medical Alert Card listed *Phenergan* as a stimulant of RLS. The card suggested *Zofran* as an acceptable alternative. This is what Jan had tried to communicate. I shared this information with the nurse, who promptly changed the medication.

Jan's mental abilities seemed to be working pretty good. On Wednesday evening I wrote the next journal entry:

> Thank you very much for the many e-mails and notes of encouragement. We plan to print them out and read to Jan as she recovers.
>
> Nurses placed a respirator tube in Jan early this morning to help calm her breathing. She is breathing much better now and we are hoping the tube can be taken out in the morning. Her blood pressure, heart rate, oxygen levels, and other vitals are now normal, except she does have a fever of 101.5 and an elevated white blood cell count.
>
> She has short periods of alertness where she is able to nod her head and point. Because of the breathing tube, we still don't know if there is any improvement with her speech. Pain levels seem to be less intense. We are not yet sure when she can be released from I.C.U. But at least for now she seems to be out of the danger zone.
>
> Assuming Jan continues to improve, our plans are

for David to drive his siblings back to Fort Worth this weekend. David will be Mr. Dad while he looks for job opportunities and the other youngins start back to their school work. I will stay here as long as Jan needs me.

While sitting with Jan today, I was thinking about Jacob and his contending with an angel, about Jeremiah who often lamented the situations he found himself in, and even Jesus in the Garden of Gethsemane. Life seems filled with adverse circumstances, especially for those who look to the Lord. But compared to the joy we will experience in eternity, "these momentary afflictions are producing for us an eternal weight of glory for beyond all comparison?" May such truths calm our aching hearts."

It was extremely frustrating for Jan not to be able to communicate. I wrote out a list of basic needs that I would read to her: Are you hot/cold? Are you in pain? Do you need to be moved? Do you need a nurse? Do you want to hear a CD?   I would read slowly until she nodded or lifted a finger. Another technique was to say each letter of the alphabet until she nodded. In this way, we could spell out key words.

The ICU had strict visiting hours: 10 a.m. to 2 p.m. and 4 p.m. to 8 p.m. The nurses were very cordial, bending the rules a bit for this mother of five. The children spent a little time with Mom each day.

However, day four saw little change in Jan's condition. She remained on a breathing machine. Her fever was over 100. Although she could respond to simple questions with a slight nod of her head, she had poor hand coordination. Her eyes could not focus. Still worst of all, she could not talk.

Fatal News

On Friday, I was finally able to talk with the ICU doctor. Standing outside Jan's room, he casually mentioned that the pathology report identified metastatic melanoma cells in Jan's brain tissue. The news hit like a rock. The hemorrhage had been caused by cancer. Jan knew that if her melanoma cancer ever reached her brain, there was almost no hope of recovery. Death often came in a matter of weeks. That's why clinical trials, with few exceptions, exclude patients with brain metastasis.

Friday, January 5, 2007:

The news today was not good. The pathology report from Jan's surgery confirmed the presence of melanoma cells in the blood and tissue. The cause of Jan's brain hemorrhage was, therefore, not AVM, but metastatic melanoma cancer. Interestingly, Jan's scans of December 8 were clear, except for her right femur bone. So we don't think the cancer is widespread. But the surgeon said that even a tiny tumor on a major blood vessel can erupt and cause severe hemorrhaging. The next step will be radiation to her head, but this cannot be done until about two weeks after surgery.

Jan would like to do the radiation in Fort Worth so she could be near the children, and Jan's surgeon thinks this is a realistic possibility. They removed Jan's breathing tube today and are evaluating her ability to breath on her own. The resident oncologist said that maybe by early next week we could evaluate the mode and timing of transporting her to Fort Worth. If she is unable to be moved, then we will do the two-week radiation treatments here in Roanoke and then transfer her at a later time.

On the positive side, Jan continues to be responsive to all questions. She can slowly nod her head, raise a finger, or signal us with a raise of her eyebrows. Though she can slowly lift her arm and flex her feet, she has no ability to hold herself up or turn her head.

Jan and I agreed long ago that full disclosure of the facts would be much better than trying to hide the truth. With the girls by her side, Jan grimaced when I shared with her the pathology report. Jan knows more than any of us what brain metastasis means. With me slowly calling out each letter of the alphabet, watching for Jan's response, Jan communicated what she wanted: H U G, and pointed toward the girls. After some long tearful hugs, the girls then sang to Mom...

God will make a way, when there seems to be
no way.   He works in ways we cannot see,
He will make a way, He will make a way.

The children will wait until Sunday morning to leave
for Fort Worth, with strong hopes that we can get Jan
to Fort Worth sooner rather than later. I will stay with
Jan. We all know that the next several weeks are going
to be difficult. But it is a great comfort to know that so
many of you are praying us through.

Saturday was a grim day. Jan and I knew that radiation
treatments would, at best, slow down the inevitable. Maybe it
could buy us a little time for her to recover some of her speech.
I wanted so much for Jan to be able to talk.

For a third time, she pointed at her white bag. She
nodded *yes* as I took out her wallet and began reading through
the calling cards. Her thumb came up when I read the name
of the doctor who had developed the dendritic vaccine used
in her clinical trial. This is the same doctor who had told her
last month that she was practically cancer free, and that his
vaccine seemed to be working well. Therefore, she didn't need
to consider any other treatment.

I smiled and said to Jan, *"You want me to write him a
letter and tell him about what you think of his vaccine?"*

Jan gave me a big smile and nodded *yes*.

Hmmm, that's Jan. In the most somber of circumstances,
she can still find something to laugh about.

I knew Sunday morning was going to be hard. The
children had to drive back to Fort Worth so they could start
their classes and school work. Jan wanted them to return to
Texas with the hope that she could soon be reunited with them.
However, it was still uncertain that Jan would ever make it back
to Texas, so the children knew this might be the last time they
ever saw their mother.

In the next journal entry, I briefly described one of the
most painful scenes I ever had to watch:

The children said a tearful goodbye this morning before they left for Texas. After some jovial conversation as Mom listened, each child, one at a time, from youngest to oldest, leaned down for a gentle hug as Mom placed her arms around and prayed silently for each one. Then, surrounding her bed, the family sang one of Jan's favorite songs...

Blessed be Your name, when I'm found in the desert place,
Though I walk through the wilderness, blessed be Your name.
Every blessing You pour out I'll turn back to praise.
When the darkness closes in, Lord, still I will say...
Blessed be the name of the Lord; blessed be Your name.
Blessed be the name of the Lord; blessed be Your
    glorious name.
Blessed be Your name, when the sun's shinning down on me,
When the world's all that it should be, blessed be Your name.
Blessed be your name, on the road marked with suffering.
Though there's pain in the offering, blessed be Your name.
You give and take away. You give and take away.
My heart will choose to say, "Lord, blessed be Your name."

When I returned to the ICU room on Sunday afternoon, I was surprised to find Jan TALKING to a visitor. The visitor was a Filipino who had worked at the International Mission Board in our Pacific Rim office. With her were her husband and two children, one (a teenage girl) had recently recovered from a severe accident

Jan's words were far from perfect, but with effort, she was making herself understood. I was elated. It was clear that her memory was sharp, because she was able to discuss some recent activities of our fellow missionaries. With effort, she was also able to speak some words of advice to the teenage daughter. Jan was more interested in talking about their situation than she was her own.

After they left, Jan was tired. But, again with effort, she shared about her hemorrhage and her trip to the emergency room. We talked a little about the children, then she had to stop. Her pain medication was taking affect and she fell asleep.

That night, I wrote:

It was a week ago on December 31st that Jan was celebrating her 50th with family and a delicious supper at Red Lobster Inn. On Dec. 11 and 12, we had visited her doctors, who assured her that there was no evidence of cancer, except a spot in her right leg. On we went to Kentucky where we stayed at a quiet Christian retreat center. Great family time.

Then we traveled over the Cumberland Gap to Virginia where we joined Jan's father, her brother's families, and her step-family. Lots of good food and family time. On Dec. 29, David, Jonathan, and I drove back to Fort Worth, expecting Jan and the girls to fly in on January 1st. Hmmm, how plans can change!

This evening Jan is doing better. She is still in ICU but her breathing is becoming less labored. There's a slight improvement in her coordination. Her fever is gone. And, for the first time in a week, she has spoken some words. Still, she has bouts of intense pain and has a long way to go before she is speaking clearly and breathing on her own.

Yesterday, I had asked Jan if she was struggling with the Lord about all of this. Without hesitation, she shook her head NO. Despite the intense pain, inability to breath, unable to speak, being mostly paralyzed, totally helpless, and having practically no hope for another birthday, Jan is letting us know that nothing will ever separate her from the hope, trust, and love she has in the Lord, Jesus Christ.

Monday morning was relatively good. For the first time, Jan swallowed a sip of water. Although her pain was intense at times, and her coughing was still frequent, her alertness and coordination were improving. She made attempts to write on a pad. I read to her the many cards and emails she had received. When she spoke, her words were mumbled, but were usually understandable.

On Monday afternoon, however, her breathing became irregular again. During the night, they had to put her back on a ventilator machine in order to calm her rapid breathing. All day Tuesday, Jan appeared exhausted from just having to breathe. I wrote that evening:

> Sunday evening and Monday were good for Jan. Her breathing had improved, words were starting to form, and even some smiles could be seen on her face. Today was not good. During the night, her breathing worsened. She had to be put back on a ventilator. Had a slight fever. No words today, no smiles. All her energy was being spent on her labored breathing.
>
> She can still nod YES or NO; can still lift a thumb or squeeze my hand. The doctor and nurses are thinking it's time for a tracheotomy – an air tube inserted through a tiny opening in the neck. But Jan has indicated that she's not ready for it just yet. I suspect she wants to give her body every chance to do the work on its own. Most of our decisions about getting her out of ICU, transporting her to Texas, and starting radiation therapy are all on hold until her breathing can be stabilized.
>
> There are other issues to confront. She can't swallow yet. For the past week she has been fed by a feeding tube through her nose. Her lungs don't have enough push to cough up mucus. She has to be suctioned. Then there's her fractured right femur bone that still causes her pain.
>
> Yet, with all this going on, her one joy is her praise music. While she is resting, and before I leave her room, I will put on one of her many worship CD's, with selections like Great Is Thy Faithfulness, Blessed Assurance, Jesus Is All The World To Me, and Moment By Moment. It is hard to imagine the depths of her thoughts during such a time as this, but I know her years of meditation in God's Word are ministering to her now. As someone has said, when the Lord is all you have, you realize He is all you need.

By Wednesday morning, Jan seemed to have regained some of her energy. They took her off the ventilator. Her breathing had stabilized. She asked about the children. I held a cell phone to her ear so the children could speak to her over the phone. At noon, one of our supervisors from the Mission Board visited us with his wife. Jan was able to say some words. To save energy, though, she communicated with as few words as possible.

After they left, Jan rested. At 2 p.m., it was time for me to leave. Jan and I shared some intimate words. As I knelt down to kiss her goodbye, she took my hand. Gently smiling, she asked me, *"You think I will die?"*

Kneeling by her bed, I drew close to her and replied, *"Well, the doctors think so. Of course, they thought so two and a half years ago. But if they are right this time, are you ready?"*

With an even bigger smile, she clearly said, *"I've been ready for a long time."*

Those were her last words to me, with all her memory and thinking intact, because that afternoon, something happened.

Another Hemorrhage

When I returned that afternoon, Jan was lethargic. She would not, or could not, talk. When she did respond, it was with a weak smile or a brief nod. I thought perhaps she was just tired, or maybe her medications were having an effect.

But when I returned the next morning and saw no improvement, I was worried. She was even less responsive. I could also detect renewed irregularity in her breathing.

After lunch, I went back to the house and wrote the following:

I just returned from the hospital where Jan is still in ICU. Let me first say thank you very, very much for all the cards and emails. I was able to read most of them to Jan on Monday, her best day so far. All the others I have read but, I'm sure you understand, haven't been able to respond.

Yesterday evening and all of today, Jan has been rather unresponsive. She will occasionally give a nod or maybe a smile, but nothing more. Her breathing is a bit erratic, but stable. Perhaps she was right about not requiring a tracheotomy. We'll see. She has no fever; her blood pressure and heart rate are good. She still cannot cough well and frequently needs to be suctioned.

The doctor shared yesterday that her alkaline phosphates and other liver enzymes have been rising over the past week. This might indicate metastatic cancer activity in the liver, but we are not sure. She still has not been able to swallow. What coordination she has is very lethargic. The pain management doctor felt it was time to discuss resuscitation issues with me, just in case.

But there is some good news. The International Mission Board has arranged medical air transport for Jan. The plan now is to fly her from Virginia to Fort Worth on Monday, where she will stay for at least a couple of days at Harris Hospital where we will evaluate what to do next. Thank you IMB!

Pray that her breathing and other vital functions will be stable enough for the transport. We are really in the dark as to what will happen to Jan physically.

What I think happened to Jan physically was subsequent hemorrhaging in other parts of her brain. A CT scan of her head confirmed a build up of cranial fluids, especially in the central ventricles. The fluids may have included new blood.

That evening, we could not wake Jan. The doctor called out to her and shook her, but no response. Her breathing was becoming more erratic and labored. We thought we were losing her.

They placed her back on a ventilator machine. We agreed that a tracheostomy (a tube inserted through her neck to her trachea – wind pipe) was necessary. The doctor scheduled the procedure for the following morning. The ventilator calmed her breathing, but Jan was still not responding. We worried through the night.

When we arrived the next morning, the trachea tube was in place. The doctor also reopened a small surgical hole at the top of her skull to drain excess cranial fluids. By the time the anesthesia wore off, Jan could open her eyes. Although she seemed a bit disoriented, she would nod her head in response to specific questions. I tried reading some recent cards and emails, but I was surprised when Jan didn't seem to recognize some of the names. She soon lost interest and wanted to sleep.

But at least she was responsive. Our hope of getting her to Texas was renewed. That Friday evening, January 12, 2007, I wrote on the website:

What a roller-coaster. Yesterday, Jan was near the bottom. Today, Jan is on the up-side. Yesterday, Jan's blood carbon dioxide levels were extremely high. Today they are close to normal range. Yesterday, Jan's breathing was very erratic and labored. Today, they surgically attached a trachea tube (a breathing tube in her neck) and her breathing is normal, though still assisted with a breathing machine.

Yesterday, a build up of cranial fluid was causing pressure on the brain. Today, a drainage hole was reopened and the pressure has subsided. Yesterday, Jan was in a coma-like condition. Today, her eyes are open and she nods her head in response to our questions.

It will be a couple of days before the trachea tube can be adjusted so that she can talk. And that's if Jan responds well to other physical factors. Her surgeon has scheduled on Monday for a permanent cranial drainage "shunt" to be placed from her head, under her skin, leading into her abdomen. A common procedure, he says, for those whose cranial fluids are unable to drain properly. This will, of course, delay her transport to Texas until later in the week.

The ICU has strict visiting hours, so I can only stay with Jan for three hours in the morning and four hours in the evening. Jan's dad has been spending time sitting with her, too. Aside from talking to the doctors and helping make Jan comfortable, there's not much for me to do while I'm there. I guess I'm not as strong as I thought; it's hard to watch her suffer like this. I often think it would make so much more sense for me to be in that bed rather than her. Her coughing / suctioning spells are especially painful to see, knowing how helpless she must feel not being able to take care of herself.

For the first time since Monday, Jan seemed alert enough for me to read some emails and cards to her. I constantly remind her of the many prayers being lifted up by all of you. Thank you so much for your love and support.

There was little change in Jan's condition the following day. The trachea tube was positioned in such a way that all air passed through the tube and none through her mouth. She couldn't speak. Although she could move her hands and feet, she wasn't smiling much. She seemed detached and contemplative, staring out the window for long periods of time.

When I arrived Sunday morning, I knew something inside of Jan had changed. Sweat was falling from her face; fear was showing in her eyes. She grabbed my arm tightly and began mouthing words of accusations against unseen people. I thought Jan's struggle was something spiritual, but now I think it was the pressure effects of cranial fluids from previous days, including possible secondary hemorrhaging. In the days to come, she would have more of these panic attacks. I would also discover that a significant part of her memory had been lost.

But I wasn't aware of these things when I wrote the next journal entry:

Jan is about the same. Still breathing on her own through the trachea tube. She occasionally has bouts of painful coughing followed by shallow breathing. Today, with lots of effort, she swallowed a little water. Her blood pressure and heart rate are still OK. No fever. Her coordination seems a bit improved. It is still too early to asses her speech abilities.

Tomorrow morning they will place a ventricular shunt from her head just behind her ear, channel it beneath her skin, and have it drain into her abdomen. The doctor is still optimistic that she should be ready to fly to Texas by Wednesday.

Well, I think I may know one reason why God allowed Jan to be in that bed instead of me. I would have wimped out. I would rather enjoy heaven than to endure this level of pain. I would have never called 911. *"Lord, take me now! Let's get this over with."* And if I did make the mistake of calling 911, I wouldn't have told them where my medical records were. The less they know, the quicker I'll go. Gosh, I probably wouldn't have bothered to keep medical records.

But, unlike me, Jan is not thinking about "I", but about you, and about her Lord. I think she wants to preserve every opportunity she has to make Christ known, even at the cost of terrible suffering. I suspect that the power of our testimony is not in the crafting of eloquent words, but in the simple, bold statements of faith spoken in the backdrop of adverse circumstances. In the past days, Jan has given us thumbs up affirmations of her dependence and trust in the Lord, Jesus Christ. And this in the midst of unspeakable pain, both physical and emotional.

Still, I don't want to presume on anything. Satan's goal is to use suffering as a wedge to separate us from God. God's goal is to use the same suffering as a means to purify our faith and lead us into a deeper fellowship with Him. While most of us can well endure a moment of suffering, there's something about persistent, unrelenting pain that surely tears at the fabric of our faith and challenges the sturdiest of souls.

Back to Texas

Jan was in surgery for about an hour and a half Monday morning. They implanted a cranial drainage tube from the back of her neck, passing downward through soft tissue, to her abdomen. Because of post-surgical pain, the nurses kept her heavily sedated throughout the day.

By Tuesday morning, Jan could open her eyes, but her attention span was short. She would occasionally lift her arm and touch the back of her head. It was still hurting. Pain medication left her drowsy most of the day.

On Tuesday evening, I wrote:

Jan will respond to our questions with a nod or an occasional smile. She opens her eyes only when we ask her to. The trachea tube prevents her from speaking. It appears she can stay focused only for a few moments before she drifts.

Yesterday morning they placed a cranial drainage "shunt" from her head to her abdomen. The surgery went well. White blood cell count still high. Also has a lot of congestion in her lungs that is painful for her to cough up. Vital signs look good. Still no fever. Also, her alkaline phosphates have been declining, meaning she may not have cancer metastasis to her liver as we previously suspected. Today, a swallowing test indicated that Jan is not yet ready to start eating or drinking.

Tomorrow, I think we are good to go. As long as Jan's condition stays stable tonight and there is a bed available at Harris Hospital in the morning, we are scheduled to leave Roanoke around lunch time in a Cessna twin engine medical transport jet.

After her arrival at the ICU of Harris Hospital in downtown Fort Worth, we will evaluate her overall physical status and see what options we have for her care. While Peggy, our resident angel, stays with Jan, I will go home to see if the kids have left the house intact.

Let me say again how much I have appreciated everyone's help. From the cards, gifts, and emails, to the ones who sent food to my youngins in Fort Worth, your labor of love has been clearly evident. Jan and I are blessed to have so many friends who care. I thank God in my remembrance of you all.

Early Wednesday morning, we received word that no beds were available at Harris Hospital. The flight transport would have to be delayed. I worked the phones, calling the hospital in Roanoke and calling offices in Fort Worth, trying to find an available oncology ward hospital bed.

With Peggy's help in Fort Worth, we found and reserved a bed at All Saints Hospital downtown. The flight was rescheduled for the following morning. At the hospital, Jan seemed to understand that she would be flying to Fort Worth where the children were. She appeared pleased and ready to go.

That afternoon, a nurse showed me how to use a trachea valve. The valve blocked the outflow of air from the tube and diverted it through her vocal cords and mouth. Although it was difficult, Jan managed to breathe some simple words, but nothing that alerted me to her impaired memory.

Soon after Bill and I returned home that evening, we received a phone call from the hospital that Jan was being moved out of the ICU and into a private room. We questioned if Jan was ready for this, but the hospital needed the ICU bed. Bill and I took turns staying with Jan through the night and the next morning. During the night she had another anxiety attack, this one lasting much longer. Not until the nurse sedated her did she relax.

The air transport team arrived at noon. They took Jan by ambulance to the Roanoke airport with Bill, Judy, and I following behind. I said my goodbyes to Bill and Judy as the transport team lifted Jan into the small Cessna jet. Aside from the pilot and co-pilot, two medical personnel sat behind me with Jan stretched out on our right side. We lifted off the runway at 1:30 on our way to Fort Worth, with a refueling stop at their headquarters in Atlanta.

In Atlanta, I got off the plane to stretch and to see their other planes. When I returned to our plane, there was activity going on inside. Jan was having another panic attack. More sedation. I was confused as to why Jan was having these attacks. Perhaps it was her medication. Maybe her CO_2 blood levels were still too high.

The plane landed in Fort Worth at 5 p.m. By 6:30, Jan was in her hospital room. Jan recognized Peggy, as well as David and Hannah when they came. With Peggy by her side, I went home to rest. Hannah wrote the next journal entry:

> Hello everyone. We just got back from the hospital
> and I'm writing this since Dad is very exhausted right
> now and just went to sleep. Let's see, Mom was supposed
> to have returned home Wednesday but Harris didn't

have a room available so their trip was delayed today. That was probably a good thing since the weather here was pretty bad so that might have caused problems in transportation once they got here.

Harris still didn't have a room available today so they decided to go to the only other hospital that has an oncology ward, Baylor All Saints. They left Roanoke around the middle of the afternoon and arrived around six-thirty this evening. Dad said the flight went relatively smoothly.

David and I came around seven-thirty to pick up Dad and their luggage. Mom smiled when we came in and greeted her but then she remained relatively quiet. It's difficult to understand what she's saying with her breathing tube and her dry mouth. She tried to talk to us but we couldn't understand a word. Compared to when us kids last saw her in Virginia she seems to have regressed a little.

She's not quite as alert and responsive as she was a week and a half ago. She can open her eyes or squeeze your hands if you ask her to but her eyes are unfocused and muscle coordination is still a problem. But when the nurse asked her to list her name, birth date, and where she was Mom was able to mouth out the correct answers to those questions.

Peggy Hodges is staying with Mom tonight and it was obvious Mom was happy to have Peggy with her. She certainly has been God's gift to us. Tomorrow, after getting some much needed rest, Dad will return to the hospital and quiz the doctor on what the next step will be for Mom.

Hopefully we'll know more tomorrow about what the near future will look like. We're working on a schedule for having someone with Mom at all times but rotating people so that no one gets burned out.

As of now Mom doesn't look like she is up to having visitors. Her attention span seems to be rather short, she'll respond or try to say something but then drift off into a kind of daze. But she seemed pretty coherent when I began the long list of describing all the different foods, dishes, and treats that people had brought over and she raised her eyebrows in amazement.

We're praying that Mom will improve and she'll be able to talk soon. Thanks so much for all the prayers and for all the people who brought over meals that have definitely added some inches around our waists! We have been overwhelmed with the generosity of so many, thank you so much! But we want to thank everyone for all the prayers being offered up for Mom right now.

A new development has been anxiety attacks. She had one this morning and then one on the plane. Dad said they seem to be something like hallucinations when she panics and loses touch with reality. The one on the plane happened when they stopped off in Atlanta to refuel. Mom became antsy and then very upset and insisted that she get off the plane because she thought she was going to die.

Please pray that Mom will not have any more anxiety attacks and that her spirit would be peaceful. I can't imagine how scary life must be for Mom right now. Please continue to pray for peace and strength. And I guess that prayer goes for all of us. I know our family has only been doing well because of the prayers of so many. God bless.

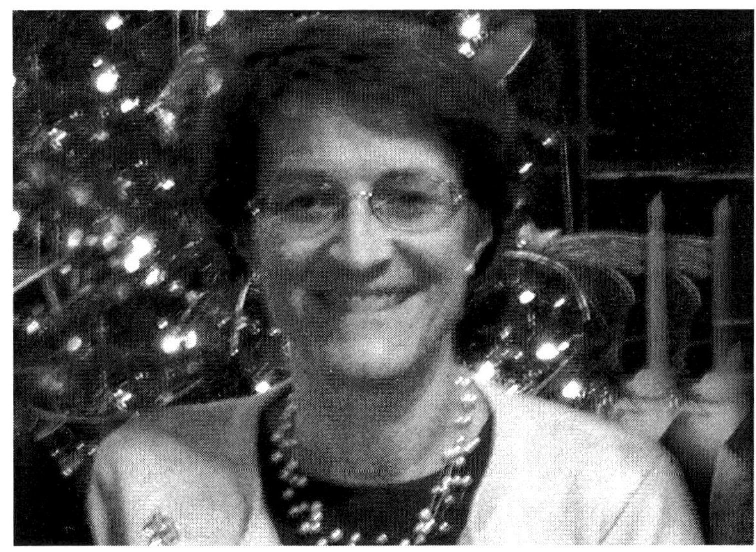

Jan - Christmas Eve 2006

Chapter 11: JAN'S PROMOTION

"Jan, how many children do you have?" I felt silly asking such an obvious question. But I was perplexed by Jan's lack of excitement when the children had visited earlier. I was also trying to find an explanation for her passive and lethargic demeanor. So, on a hunch, I asked the question. Moments passed before Jan responded.

She lifted four fingers.

My heart sank. *"Jan, can you name them?"*

The trachea tube had been adjusted so some air could pass through her vocal cords. With effort, Jan breathed out the names, *"David..., Sara..., Hannah..."* Then she stopped.

After a few moments, I asked another question, *"Jan, do you know the country we lived in for twenty years?"*

A long pause, then she shook her head *no.*

My next question, *"Jan, do you know where you are?"*

Slowly, she breathed, *"Hospital...Fort Worth."*

Of course, we had been telling her this for a couple of days. I continued, *"Do you know why you are here?"*

Another long pause, then she shook her head *no.*

It was Sunday afternoon, January 21, 2007. Peggy had stayed with Jan through the night and into the morning. I came after attending worship with the children. On Saturday, Jan had experienced another panic attack and for a while didn't know where she was. After she recovered, I had asked her if she knew why she was in the hospital. She nodded *yes* but didn't mention the word cancer. I assumed she knew. Early Sunday morning, I had written an update:

Jan is slowly recovering. The past two days, she has begun to speak words. It takes a lot of effort, though, because of the trachea tube. She is asking questions and will sometimes give us a smile. She understands her physical condition and her prognosis. Pain is still a big issue. Her medications seem to cause an occasional hallucination and some short-term memory loss. The hospital has a team of physical therapists who have begun to work with her. So far, she has been unable to sit up. On Monday, she will have a feeding tube placed through her abdomen.

Also on Monday, she will begin two and a half weeks of radiation treatments. The oncologist says these will be palliative, not curative. In other words, the aim is to alleviate pain and discomfort, and give her as many good days as we can. She will remain in the hospital for the duration of the treatments and for physical therapy. Afterwards, depending on her mobility, we will either take her to a hospice center, or to Peggy's home with hospice aid.

At this point, we still want to limit visitors until Jan is more stable and can communicate better. Peggy is keeping a schedule of qualified ladies who can be with her around the clock. I plan to be with Jan every morning from 8 to 12. That's when doctors come and decisions need to be made. This will give me time to take care of family and household needs in the afternoon and evenings. So much to be done. The children have spent some time with Mom and are handling things quite well. We have had family times where we share our feelings and how we are dealing with the stress.

We aim to see God's hand in every situation. We

remind ourselves why suffering exists. God did not cause this cancer, but He can and will use it for Jan's eternal benefit and for our spiritual growth. Without suffering, we would never recognize happiness. Without pain, we would never understand peace. Adversity contrasts with joy, and helps us define it. Hardships remind us that earth is not our home. Martha wrote a poem the other day and expressed it this way:

You don't value what you have, 'til you have to do without,
you don't value the rain, 'til you live through a drought.
You don't value light, 'til you're trapped in the dark,
you don't value peace, 'til war has left its mark.
You don't value a home, 'til you wander, nowhere to be,
you don't value sight, 'til it's black and cannot see.
You don't value sound, 'til silence, you cannot hear,
you don't value fellowship, 'til you're lonely, no one near.
You don't value warmth, 'til you're shivering in the cold,
you don't value nature, 'til there's no beauty to behold.
You don't value a breeze, 'til you're sweating in the heat,
you don't value joy, 'til sorrow has you beat.
You don't value family, 'til they're beneath the earth to stay,
you don't value life, 'til you feel it slip away.

Martha understood, as did the rest of us, that Jan's time was short. However, we were hoping Jan could recover some of her speaking ability and experience better days ahead.

But now, on Sunday afternoon, there was a bigger issue. In addition to Jan's speech, was there any chance she could regain her memory and mental capacity? It would be another ten days before any medical personnel would risk an answer. Until then, we hoped.

No Improvement

On Tuesday evening, I wrote:

Advance Directives. Medical Power of Attorney. Out-of-Hospital Do-Not-Resuscitate Order. These are some of the terms that have been presented to me this week. Jan's long-term condition doesn't look good. She still breaths through her trachea tube, which also hinders her attempts to speak. Because of sedation, she hasn't progressed much with physical therapy. A lung infection still gives her coughing spells. She's being fed through a stomach tube.

Worst of all, she has a degree of amnesia. Immediately after her hemorrhage on January 1, and for the next 10 days, Jan's memory was fine, even describing events surrounding her emergency trip to the hospital.

But around the 11th and 12th, a CT scan showed swelling in her brain ventricles, which led to the implanting of a cranial drainage shunt. Since then, her memory and reasoning abilities haven't been good. She has moments of disorientation and confusion.

Jan and I used to talk about what we would do in this kind of situation. Her desire was that if there was a reasonable chance for her to recover her mental abilities and have some good days, then she would want everything done to keep her alive. So this is what I will do.

She began radiation treatments today. Speech and physical therapy will continue. Still, doctors caution that Jan is in a delicate condition and anything could happen, such as another hemorrhage.

It is during times such as these that God's truths provide a firm anchor for my wavering emotions. I have learned that sickness and suffering are consequences of man's sinfulness, and that these same trials can be motivations to cry out to God (Psalm 50:15), reminders of our weaknesses (2 Corinthians 12: 7-10), preparations to comfort others (2 Corinthians 1: 3-5), methods of purifying our faith (1 Peter 1: 6-7), and ways of increasing our hatred for evil (Proverbs 8:13).

Jan understood all of this and was able to put her physical hardships in eternal perspective, knowing that her *momentary affliction is producing for us an eternal weight of glory far beyond all comparison* (2 Corinthians 4:17). I believe it is this *living hope* (1 Peter 1:3) that is carrying Jan through each day, and it will carry us, too.

Back at home, Jonathan had started back to his Tuesday / Thursday school. Martha struggled to stay focused on her studies. Hannah resumed her studies where she had left off in December. Sara was back in her college classes. David was helping out where he could. The children visited Jan almost every day, occasionally staying several hours. Peggy stayed with Jan each night until I came in the morning. Different ladies volunteered to stay with Jan in the afternoon and evening hours.

But Jan was not improving. Friday the 26th was my next journal entry:

Jan is about the same. On the positive side, her breathing, via the trachea tube, is good. Her lung congestion has lessened. No fever. Her morphine drip has made her comfortable; no intense pain.

She is getting specialized food in her stomach via a feeding tube. The nurses are taking good care of her. Peggy has been keeping a schedule so that someone is with her around the clock (thank you, ladies, very very much!).

On the negative side, her memory is still not good. There are some major things she cannot remember, and this is frustrating for her. When I place a trachea valve over her tube, she is able to speak some words for short periods.

It is still difficult for her to focus, so she keeps her eyes closed. She has been too sedated to do any physical therapy. But she does give a smile when people greet her and a gentle wave of her hand when they leave.

She finished her first week of radiation treatments today; another six treatments to go. They sedate her before each treatment in order to lessen any chance of anxiety. Please pray with us about where to take Jan after her treatments are done. There are several options: rehabilitation unit, skilled nursing care, hospice unit, or home care. All depends on the doctor's recommendations and Jan's condition.

Let me take this chance to again express my deep appreciation for all your words of encouragement through cards, emails, and the postings on this guestbook. All praise goes to the Lord, Jesus Christ who gives His grace for the moment and His promises for eternity.

The weekend was disappointing as we saw no improvement in Jan's condition. Still, we hoped the radiation treatments would buy her a little more time to improve. David's last college term would start the first of February; he would leave on Tuesday. We made an effort that weekend to spend extra time with David, and David spent extra time with Mom.

Knowing it was doubtful Jan would ever return to the house, I began to sort through the things in her room. On Monday evening, I wrote:

I have spent a little time this week going through Jan's papers, looking for medical information. In the process, I've come across several of her devotional books and notes.

When we wonder how a person like Jan can expound and apply God's Word so relevantly to life's situations, look no further than her chair and bedside. There, next to her Bibles, I've found notes and notebooks journaling her walk with the Lord. Here are some verses, written on note cards, that she was working on hiding in her heart...

1 Peter 5:10 *"In his kindness God called you to His eternal glory by means of Jesus Christ. After you have suffered a little while, He will restore, support, and strengthen you, and He will place you on a firm foundation."*

Hebrews 6: 11-12 *"We want each of you to show this same diligence to the very end, in order to make your hope sure. We do not want you to become sluggish, but to imitate those who through faith and patience inherit what has been promised."*

Philippians 1: 20-21 *"I eagerly expect and hope that I will in no way be ashamed, but will have sufficient courage so that now as always Christ will be exalted in my body, whether by life or by death. For me to live is Christ and to die is gain."*

Jan starts another week of radiation treatments. Her vital signs remain stable, but she continues to receive medications, including a steady morphine drip to manage her pain. An infection has developed in front of her left ear. Antibiotics are being given. She hasn't been able to get out of bed for 29 days. Can't even sit up. Much of her memory is still gone. She's been too sedated to do any physical therapy. She's only been given small amounts of food through her feeding tube because it just isn't being digested well. In short, her body is not recovering.

But she can still smile. My hope is that God's Word, hidden in her heart, is finding ways to minister to her spirit.

Transfer to Hospice

David wanted to stay, but I encouraged him to return to college, knowing this would be Jan's wish, too. On Tuesday morning, he packed his car (the one we bought on December 31). On his way out, he dropped by the hospital for a final visit.

I told him that a hospital specialist wanted to talk with me later that morning. While we still held on to a tiny hope that Jan would recover some of her abilities, David knew that this was likely the last time he would see his mother. Jan had her eyes open but wasn't moving her arms or legs. She could hear but was making no attempts to speak. I allowed David some private moments with Mom. He talked with her, prayed, and said goodbye.

About thirty minutes after David left, I sat in a waiting room with the specialist and the hospital chaplain. The specialist explained that Jan's team of doctors and nurses had concluded that there was nothing more they could do for Jan. She was not responding to any therapy. Her food, administered through a stomach tube, was not digesting. It seemed her body systems were slowly shutting down.

I asked if there was any chance she might regain some of her memory and speech. The specialist said that seldom does a patient in Jan's condition see any improvement in their mental abilities. On rare occasions, a patient may experience some memory restoration during their final days, due in part by reduced cranial pressure caused by dehydration. But this, she again cautioned, was rare.

So, the time had come for Jan to make the transition from hospital to Hospice care. The purpose of a hospital is to do all they can medically to keep a patient alive and help him improve. The purpose of Hospice is to provide a comfortable and dignified exit. With Peggy's help, we made arrangements with a Hospice care facility in Fort Worth. A bed would be available on Friday.

On Thursday afternoon, February 1, 2007, I entered the next update:

I just returned from the hospital where Jan is resting well and is comfortable. It seems that we have arrived at that dreaded day. Jan's team of doctors has concluded that there is nothing more they can do for her. All indications are that Jan's body is slowly shutting down. None of her food is digesting. Her movements are slower. She is constantly tired.

Tomorrow afternoon we will transfer her to Community Hospice of Texas, whose focus is comfort care. She will be at 1111 Summit Ave. for a few days until we can hopefully transfer her to Peggy's house. Starting Saturday, short visits will be okay. Their assessment of Jan's condition is that her time is more likely measured in days rather than weeks.

So, it's time to end the doctor visits, the scans, the medications, the treatments, the clinical trials, and the research. It's time to accept that these are the days God has ordained for Jan since before she was born (Psalm 139). We knew the time would come, but didn't want to think about the emotions that would come with it. They could wait to be dealt with on a distant day. Now that day has come. And it's not easy....

But with the grief, we find reasons to rejoice. Jan has finished her race (2 Timothy 4:7), she has kept her faith. She has let it shine. Now there is in store for her the rewards God has promised in accordance with her service and faith. And she will soon be able to enjoy those for eternity.

I've been going through some of the video tapes we have of Jan that others have recorded for us. Here, Jan remembers the day nearly three years ago when the doctor told her that the cancer had spread:

"I had been reading in the Psalms where it says that "the righteous will have no fear of bad news. His heart is steadfast. He will not be shaken, because He trusts in You." So when the physician called and said, "I've got bad news: the cancer is in the lymph nodes." And I said, "You know, I'm not surprised. And God is not surprised." You know, bad news doesn't have to rattle me. I come back to the sovereignty of God. I know God is in control."

On Friday morning, I explained to Jan where we were going. I'm not sure she understood, but neither did she object. She was sedated prior to the trip to avoid anxiety. An ambulance transferred her to the Hospice center, just a short distance from the hospital. Her room was a quiet relief from the busyness of the hospital. The staff was exceptional. Almost immediately, Jan seemed more relaxed and at peace. She never had any more anxiety attacks.

My next update was on Saturday afternoon:

Jan's room at the Hospice Center is large and restful. It's carpeted. There's a sofa and a recliner. Her window overlooks downtown Fort Worth. The nurses are friendly, sympathetic, and eager to help. Our Number One nurse and friend, Peggy, stays with Jan through the night. I left there about an hour ago and Jan seems comfortable. She still occasionally opens her eyes, can mouth a few words, respond to questions with a nod, and still manage a bit of a smile. But there are other signs that show us her transition is near. We probably won't make it to Peggy's house.

The children were with her this morning. They talked and sang to her. This is a transition time for them, too. Some are struggling through it more than others. They all are having to grow up a little faster.

Last night we stayed up late planning for the memorial service. There was both laughter and sadness as we sorted through piles of pictures. On a video segment, Jan shared this:

"Let me tell you about the valedictorian of our High School class... This person was voted most likely to succeed. Best in science and math. ...and had all these awards... 30 years later, that person doesn't own a car, doesn't own a house, no big salary, nobody probably knows much about this person. Is this person successful? Has this person accomplished anything? In the world's eyes probably not. But that person is me.

Maybe in the world's eyes I haven't been successful. But, I thank God for the life we've had, because it's been a good one. If we're doing what God wants us to do, we don't have to worry about being successful. We're just being faithful. That's what I want to hear when I go to heaven, is God saying, "Well done, my good and faithful servant." He doesn't say, "My good and successful servant." I may have not accomplished much in the world's eyes, but the One I'm concerned about pleasing is Him, so that's okay."

Back in 2005, some family friends had the idea to do a video taped interview with Jan. My brother, Steve, was thinking of this, too. So in December of 2005, just a couple of weeks apart, Jan conducted two, 1½ hour interviews. Now I began making preparations to include portions of these interviews in Jan's Memorial Service. We cherished her words.

Final Days

With Jan now in Hospice care, Bill and Judy began the long journey from Virginia to Fort Worth. Jan had a large number of visitors on Sunday afternoon. She would respond with smiles and nods, occasionally mouthing a few words. At one point, she asked if Jonathan was eating too much sugar.

There were other indications that she had regained some of her memory. Overall, it was a relatively good day.

But on Monday, she was much less responsive. I wrote:

Jan had lots of visitors this weekend. She was somewhat alert, able to open her eyes and smile occasionally. On Saturday, I shared with her our plans for the Memorial Service. She smiled, nodded her head, and seemed pleased. We read Scripture to her and talked about heaven.

But today she is much weaker. No strength in her arms; no grip to her hands. Only a few times did she try to open her eyes. No nods. No smiles. I don't think she has the strength for it. But she has a peace about her and I know she is comfortable. She's ready to go. Her Dad and step-mother arrived this afternoon. Before I left the hospital, I prayed with Jan, releasing her into the Lord's hands.

Tomorrow is Hannah's birthday. She will be the first to open her birthday card from Mom, one of many that Jan wrote last year to each of the children for the next several years. Tonight, we will work on the Memorial Service. Let me share with you some more of Jan's words that were recorded on video:

"A lot of people ask the question, "Why did you get cancer?" Of course, Mark and I answer, "Why not"? One out of every three Americans get it; we just decided to do it at the same time... But it's important to know that God is in control. He allows things to happen in our lives, He doesn't cause them. He didn't cause this cancer. When I found out about Mark, my question to God was, "Are you sure You can trust us this much?"

"Because nothing happens to us that He has not allowed to happen. Scripture says, He will not tempt us beyond what we are able to handle. We can handle anything through Him. So, He must really trust us. It was almost like an honor. He trusted us enough to allow this. So, then, our response needed to be, what then do we do with this. And it has been our prayer all along that God would be glorified in it."

We felt Jan might go at anytime. So we made a decision to spend some time with her as a family that night. Shortly after sunset, we gathered in her room. While we talked and sang, we saw slight movements of her head that told us she could still hear. I wanted each child to have some private moments with Mom to say whatever they wanted to. So beginning with Jonathan, each one spent about ten minutes with Mom, while the rest of us waited outside her room. By the time I went in, her pillow was wet.

Although the day of one's homegoing to heaven is a cause for both grief and celebration, we didn't really want Jan's homegoing to occur on Hannah's birthday. So we worried a bit when Jan was still unresponsive on Tuesday morning. But by Tuesday afternoon, she began to stir. Hannah was treated to a birthday dinner by her friends. Later, she opened her card from Mom. The front of the card read...

Happy Birthday precious daughter... thank you for being one of the sweetest blessings God has given... thank you for bringing so much love and joy to my life... thank your for showing how wonderful God is by expressing how beautiful He is in you.

On Wednesday morning, I called Peggy for an update, then wrote on the website:

Well, Jan is still with us. I just talked to Peggy on the phone and she said Jan had a good night. Let me give you a run down of what has happened.

On Monday, Jan was not responding much at all. So, on Monday night, while it was quiet, I brought the children (minus David, who is at college) to the hospice center. Each of us had a private time with Jan to talk with her and say our goodbyes. I think we went through a whole box of tissues. We even saw tears on Jan's face. We sang some songs, prayed, then released her into the Lord's hands.

On Tuesday morning, Jan was not responding at all. She began having episodes of erratic breathing. Then, in the afternoon, she began to respond by briefly opening her eyes and giving an occasional smile. She even nodded in response to questions. This gave Hannah peace of mind to enjoy a great birthday celebration with family and friends. As we left her last night, with more friends visiting her and staying by her bedside, Jan was still responding.

Peggy said that this morning, Jan would still partially open her eyes, give a small smile, even lifted her hand at one point. Her blood pressure is good, lungs sound clear. But her heart rate is fast, and her breathing is still somewhat erratic. The hospice nurses, who have a lot of experience observing patients in the dying process, say that it's not unusual for a patient to be near death, then briefly recover, and maybe do this cycle for a few times, before the final moments. Still, they caution, things could happen quickly.

So, we will just wait and allow God to determine the moment. When it comes, our plans are to have a closed casket public visitation at Thompson's, Harveson, & Cole at 702 8th Ave. Then we would have a private family time, followed by the burial. The Memorial Service would follow. Let me take this opportunity to say again what a tremendous encouragement all of you have been. We appreciate so much your emails, cards, and postings on this guestbook. It is because of you that the Lord is free to work in us.

Jan could give a little nod or smile, enough to show us she could still hear. I asked her if she was having any pain? She indicated *no*. Was she at peace? She nodded *yes*. With Peggy by her side, I left to work on burial and Memorial Service preparations. Bill and Judy also continued to stay, with Jan's older brother and his wife making visits when they could.

Jan's Homegoing

On Wednesday night, I attended the prayer service of Birchman Baptist Church, where the Memorial Service would be held. Jan and I were married here twenty three years ago.

We still considered it our home church. They had a special time of prayer for Jan. But I was especially touched when an older friend expressed a desire to end the service with a prayer for my family. Through it, the Lord ministered to me.

I woke early Thursday morning with nausea and a fever. With Jan's condition about the same, I stayed home to work on my part of the Memorial Service. The girls visited with her in the afternoon, along with a group of ladies from the church. When asked to smile for the ladies, Jan did so.

In the evening, I needed to pick up a DVD for the Memorial Service. Just before I left the house, Peggy called from the Hospice center, explaining that Jan's breathing was deteriorating. The girls decided to go to the center. Jonathan didn't feel like he wanted to see Mom again in this condition, and that was okay. The girls left with two friends from the church, while I went to pick up the DVD.

It was 9 p.m. by the time I arrived at the center. Bill and Judy were there, along with the girls and their two friends. Peggy was by her side. It was obvious Jan was in her final hours. Her breathing was heavy and labored; her face sunken and her feet cold. For the next two hours, we surrounded her with songs, Scripture readings, and words of love.

So many thoughts ran through my mind, so many feelings touched my heart. I remembered when we first met, our courting days, our first year of marriage, and the day David was born. I recalled some of our times together on the mission field, and the first days of our cancer adventure. It was hard to believe her time had now come. Oh, how I wished it had been me on this bed instead of her.

We were all quiet for a few moments after Jan offered up her last breath. At about 11 p.m., the nurse checked for a pulse and recorded her pronouncement. We slowly made our way out into the waiting room while the nurse removed Jan's tubes and straightened up the bed. I called David.

It was 1 a.m. when we arrived home. With a heavy heart, I added the next entry:

Jan was promoted into the Lord's presence at 11 pm Thursday evening. The girls, Peggy, Jan's father, step-mother, brother, and some close friends from the church were all there. We read Scripture, sang songs, and encouraged her on. She left this world peacefully. Her journey over. Her joy made complete.

We will have visitation at the funeral home from 2 to 5 on Sunday afternoon. The family will have a private burial on Monday morning. This is as Jan wished. Then the Memorial Service will be at 4 pm Monday afternoon, at Birchman Baptist Church, 9100 N. Normondale.

The Memorial Service will be a celebration of a life well lived. We will be wearing white or light colors, as Jan requested. We will have music, sharing, pictures, and video clips of Jan. In speaking about the Memorial Service, Jan had this to say:

"There will be people there who don't understand... Why would God let ya'll have cancer, let ya'll suffer... I don't think we could go through any of this without believing in and trusting in the sovereignty of God. We believe what God's Word says about Him, that He is sovereign and He's in control.

And He's got this big, worldwide, eternal focus that we, as finite human beings, don't have. And He knows what He's wanting to do, in the lives, not just in our family, but other people's lives around the world. And if He can use any of this to bring one person into His kingdom, it's worth it.

I know where I'm going; I don't mind dying... I have a place I'm going to... But it's those people that don't know Him; I don't see how anyone gets thru something like this without knowing the Lord. And that's what I would encourage people there at the service... to accept Him as their Lord and Savior. That's the only thing worth living for in life, and that's following Him."

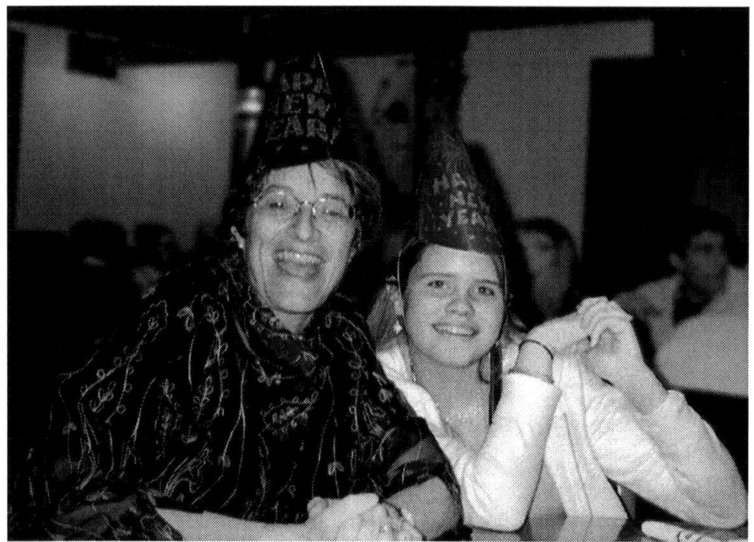

Jan (with Martha) celebrating her 50th birthday - December 31, 2006

Chapter 12: HER TESTIMONY CONTINUES

With most of the arrangements for the Memorial Service in place, we spent that weekend with each other, walking through our emotions...

Sadness. Mom was gone. We all knew the time was coming; we all knew it was inevitable. Still, the finality of her absence hit hard. Each of us had our crying moments.

Relief. Her misery was over. It pained us to see Jan suffer; to see her unable to move and communicate. Now she was free from these restraints.

Gladness. She was in heaven. We talked about all the things Mom was probably doing in heaven. And we knew that someday we would be there with her.

Gratefulness. We were overwhelmed by people's expressions of love and concern through prayers, words of encouragement, and gifts. We were blessed.

Weeks earlier, Jonathan and Hannah had signed up to serve at our church's Valentines Day Banquet on that Friday evening. Certainly folks would understand if they didn't show up. But the kids decided to keep their commitment, knowing the activity would be good for them. So, less than 24 hours after their Mom had been promoted, Jonathan and Hannah spent the evening serving food and cleaning tables at the church.

After the banquet, Hannah and I stayed to enjoy the Valentines Day program in the church sanctuary. The organizers, Martin and Shirley Coleman, dedicated the evening in Jan's honor. Again, we were blessed.

David arrived Friday night from Tennessee. On Saturday, I finalized the last of the burial and Memorial Service arrangements. Sara went to the funeral home with Judy and Jan's sister-in-law (Eva) to decorate the receiving room. In the evening, the family enjoyed a delicious meal at Peggy's house prepared by caring people. That night, I posted the next update:

It's been a busy day. Lots of time with family and friends. Lots of food. People are so kind. David arrived yesterday from Tennessee. Tonight, I told David that right now, it doesn't yet seem real. It seems that Jan will walk into the room anytime. But in the following days, weeks, and months, there will be moments of grief, when the permanency of Jan's earthly absence will be painfully real. David agreed.

Tomorrow morning, we will be in worship. In the afternoon, from 2 to 5, we will be at the funeral home. Monday morning, the family will bury Jan's "shell". The Memorial Service will be 4 pm in the afternoon at Birchman Baptist Church (9100 N. Normondale). I will lead the service (pray for me, please). The children will have a part. Along with songs and sharing, we will have a 10 minute video presentation of Jan's life, and 12 minutes of video clips of Jan sharing about cancer, death, and life. Here's another portion of what she will share:

"Maybe you've heard me share this story about my Mom... About six months after she died, David and Sara were playing, and they were so cute. I remember thinking, as I had many times in that six months, "If only Mom were here." And God just stopped me and

said, "You know, if your Mom were here, these things would bring her pleasure, they would bring her joy to see her grandchildren playing like this. But, the glories here in heaven are nothing compared to what we have on earth.

So whatever brings the greatest joy on earth is nothing compared to what will bring us joy in heaven... Like what my Mom said in a letter that was read at her funeral service, not to be sad for her... And, I think I have encouraged my children that it's OK to grieve. Scripture says, "We grieve, but not as those who have no hope." And that is one thing that Martha has said has given her hope in knowing that she will see me again."

Bill, Judy, Jan's brothers and their families joined us for Sunday morning worship. After lunch, we drove to the funeral home. For three hours we enjoyed a reunion of family and friends. I was especially honored by the presence of so many missionaries and representatives from the International Mission Board, including its President, Dr. Jerry Rankin, who had twice visited our home years ago in the Philippines when he was our Area Director.

By Jan's prior request, the casket remained closed. Flowers decorated the walls, as well as pictures from Jan's past. The large room was crowded with friends, some of whom had traveled from as far as Georgia and Tennessee. One of the funeral home employees commented that the lively atmosphere in the receiving room was more like a wedding reception than a funeral. Jan would have loved it.

That evening we rested in preparation for the busy tomorrow.

Burial and Memorial Service

Morning rain was falling when we arrived at the funeral home. The children, Jan's family, my brother and his family, gathered in the receiving room. This time, by Jan's prior request, the casket was opened. There was no program or service, just a time for us to talk about Jan and share our feelings, to give her a final touch; to whisper a last goodbye. Of course, we knew it was just her *shell*, but what a precious *shell* it had been.

After an hour, we left the funeral home and followed the hearse to the cemetery. We crowded under the canopy to shield ourselves from the drizzling rain. Again, there was no program or service. I simply said a few words, read a Scripture passage, and offered a prayer in memory of Jan – a faithful wife, a godly mother, a loving daughter, a delightful sister, and a wonderful friend to many.

As I wiped away a tear, I also smiled to myself, remembering the moment months earlier when Jan stood on this very spot, laughing at the thought of looking upon this burial *plot* while her brother was out looking for a house *lot*. I think now, in her *lot* in heaven and in God's presence, she is laughing with joy.

The church sanctuary was crowded and I was nervous as we made final preparations for the Memorial Service. I had conducted my mother's funeral years earlier, and that had been hard. I had no idea if I could make it through this. But I had offered to lead it and Jan had agreed.

In the last two Caringbridge journal entries, I described the Memorial Service:

> The children and I opened the service with a bang (party bottle poppers) as we shouted, *"It's Mom's year of Jubilee; she's happy now and forever free!"* Each read some of Jan's favorite Scriptures and gave an affirmation of Mom. All of us recited her theme Scripture – Isaiah 43: 1-3.
>
> We watched a 10 minute slide/video presentation of Jan's life. Jan concluded with the example of the peanut. *"When you take a peanut, what remains is the shell. You throw it away. The real me, who I am, the essence of Jan, has gone on to be with the Lord in heaven. This body here is just the shell, but the NUT has gone on ahead."*
>
> I expressed appreciation for all who ministered to us during our cancer adventure, but especially

appreciated Peggy Hodges long labor of love, and the International Mission Board's faithful support. I also introduced Selah Helms and Bro. Miles Seaborn who both spoke affirmingly and affectionately of Jan. Jan's step-mother, Judy Joness, sang a special number in Jan's honor.

We watched a 5 minute video of Jan explaining her favorite song, Blessed Be Your Name. The song expressed Jan's commitment to bless the Lord regardless of her circumstances. Shirley Coleman led us in singing the song with Karyn Laing at the piano.

Next, we watched a 12 minute video of Jan talking about her life, cancer, death, and eternity. Most of what she said I have already posted in the past five updates. Following the video, I gave a 15 minute eulogy, which I'll summarize below. Martha then read her poem, Shirley Coleman sang Find Us Faithful, and Bro. Bob Pearl of Birchman Baptist Church, closed the service with prayer.

"When I first met Jan, she had curly hair, a big smile, and a bounce that reminded me of Tigger, the jovial Winnie the Pooh character. But she was passionately serious about her relationship with the Lord, Jesus Christ.

It didn't take me long to realize that she could have been almost anything. With a B.S. in Biology from UVA, she could have gone on to become a doctor. Her medical knowledge always amazed me. She could have been a college professor. She could develop curriculum and teach five grade levels at one time. She could have been a public relations officer. She could listen well and talk to anyone. I think she could have won the Science Nobel Peace Prize she dreamed of while in High School. On the other hand, I think she would have made a great circus clown.

But she chose to answer God's call to be a missionary. It was this calling that God used to bring us together. We were married here at Birchman on Dec. 31, 1983, appointed to the Foreign Mission Board in Dec. of 1985, and began 19 years of wonderful ministry on the Philippine island of Panay. Jan was a mother, teacher, counselor, WMU advisor, assistant church planter, and a friend to many. But I think most people enjoyed Jan because she would make them laugh. There was never enough time around the dinner table to listen to all of her stories.

Jan was instrumental in the salvation of hundreds. Through her prayers and witness, she contributed to the spiritual growth of thousands. She was a partner in the planting and growing of many churches in the Philippines. During the past three years, we have received hundreds of letters and notes from friends in the Philippines, many who would be here today if they could. (I then read a letter from one of our co-workers written in May of 2005, where she said, *"Jan, always remember that there are many people here in the Philippines whose lives you have touched."*).

Jan and I didn't answer God's call to missions reluctantly. We didn't feel forced into it. We never felt it was a sacrifice. We became missionaries for *"the joy set before us."* The joy of being on the front line of missions and partnering with God Himself in redeeming a lost world. The joy of seeing lives transformed by the power of the Holy Spirit.

What do you think Jan would have said to God, if, 21 years ago, God would have told Jan, *"Jan, I want you to sign on to be my missionary to the Philippines. It will be hot and sweaty. You will have to live for a time in a tiny apartment with no running water. You will have to move your family and belongings more than 15 times. You will experience malaria, dengue fever, typhoid, and amoebic dysentery. Then, you will suffer for three years with terminal cancer."*

What do you think Jan would have said?

Jan, whose number one goal was to bring glory to God; who understood just how much God, through Jesus Christ, had forgiven her for her sins; whose desire in life was not to have a big house, a comfortable life, or financial security; who understood God's purposes for suffering; who knew that the means by which suffering comes doesn't matter near as much as our response when in the midst of it; whose heart-dream was to hear Jesus tell her in heaven, *"Well done, my good and faithful servant, enter into the joy of your master."*

What do you think Jan would have said to God?

I know exactly what Jan would have said, *"Lord, sign me up."* Jan would have none of us think that somehow she was deprived of anything here on earth. Indeed, Jan experienced a joy that few people ever find. Now she has eternity to enjoy the rewards of her faith and service. Jan would gladly say, *"It was well worth going through the suffering, to have what I have now."*

Jan is more alive now than she ever was here on earth. She has no more cancer, pain, or sorrow. She is free forever from the entanglement of sin. She is free from disease, aging, and hurt. She has more joy in God's presence than anything this world could ever offer. As she was fond of quoting, *"Eye has not seen, ear has not heard, mind has not conceived of all the Lord has in store for those who love Him."* Jan also has the joy of knowing all her children will share eternity with her.

On January 11, Jan experienced a subsequent swelling in the ventricles of her brain. Much of her thinking and memory was affected. But on January 10, while still in ICU, Jan had asked me, *"Mark, do you think I'm going to die."* I told her that the doctors think so, but that they had thought so two years ago. Jan smiled. I then said, *"Jan, if the doctors are right this time, are you ready to go."* With an even bigger smile, she said, *"I've been ready for a long time."* Those were her last words to me, with all her thinking and memory intact.

Jan was one of the most intelligent persons I've ever known. She used that intelligence to study God's word, to minister in God's kingdom. But it wasn't her intelligence that brought her into a relationship with the Lord. In her last year of college, she made the step of faith that God requires for anyone to know Him personally and intimately. From then on, Jan experienced God's love in her life, His power on her life, and His joy flowing through her life, to you and me."

Aside from her goal of giving glory to God, Jan's most important legacy was in the lives of her children. I was very proud of Martha for verbalizing her feelings in a poem at the end of the Memorial Service. I'll close this entry with her words:

I look but I cannot find you
I search but your spirit has gone.
I know this is not your life's evening
It's really only your dawn.

Your soul is praising in heaven
It's dancing in paradise.
Though your shell is lifeless and still
And your hand as cold as ice.

My heart is crying, weeping
My eyes beckoning tears.
I long for times past
To walk back through the years.

Never again will you comfort me
Never will you hold me tight.
You've left me stranded in darkness
While you're running toward the light.

I knew this time would come
When cancer began to seep.
It was the lighting before the thunder
But the thunder still shakes me deep.

I love you so much, Mother
It hurts me to have you go.
I want to be strong for you
Though my spirit is so low.

But I thank my Savior, my God
For giving Jesus, His Son.
So you may live eternally
That death has not quite won.

We were always moving so much
Hard to find a place to stay.
But now you've moved for the last time
To your real home far away.

It's hard to let you go
But I know that now you're free.
No hurt, no fear can hold you down
Jesus is your Jubilee.

Oh, thank you, for giving to the Lord
Because of you, I'll never be the same.
You've touched so many lives
You've brought glory to His name.

I pray your testimony won't end
Though you now walk on streets of gold.
I praise the Lord for the peace
That you so faithfully told.

It was worth to suffer trials
To have God walk with me.
And He is living over death
A glorious victory.

We grieve and weep our loss
Of a mother, wife, sister, and friend.
A crushed, a broken heart we have
But there is One who can mend.

Run to the Redeemer
for He's always there.
Ask of the Lord
Only He can repair.

At times I feel strong
During others, near despair.
But God is the one that heals the broken
He renews the heart that tears.

Mother, I must now say farewell
For in our Savior's presence you dwell.
I'll greet you again, one joyful day,
In heaven above, for eternity's stay.

Words of Hope

In one of the last Caringbridge journal entries, I wrote:

"It honored the Lord." That was the comment after the Memorial Service I liked hearing the most, because that was the goal Jan wanted. With nearly 500 in attendance, we were especially honored by the presence of Bro. Jerry Rankin, president of our International Mission Board, and the presence of other IMB personnel and fellow missionaries. There were folks from Gray, Georgia, where Jan once worked on a wildlife refuge. Several who knew Jan drove up from Houston. Others came from Oklahoma, Arkansas and Tennessee. Overall, it was quite a reunion of friends that Jan would have loved.

Several were asking about the kids and our future plans. David will be graduating in May from Union University in Tennessee with a computer science degree. He already has been hired by Datatel, Inc., the Fairfax, Virginia company where he interned last summer. We had hoped for a job here in Fort Worth / Dallas area, but this seems to be the best opportunity for David at this time. He will spend a month with us this summer before reporting to work in mid June. We are so very proud of David.

Sara is in her second semester at Tarrant County College pursuing a degree in graphic communications. Has all A's so far and really enjoys her courses. She'll be entering the job world after she graduates in May of next year. It has been exciting to see all the neat projects she has developed using her artistic talents. Jan was so very pleased for Sara to find an area where she could really excel.

Hannah is finishing her junior year of High School (although she has already received some college course credits). Her goal is to have enough college credits by the summer of next year to enter college as a 2nd year student. She scored really high on her SAT college entrance exam and will have no problem getting an academic scholarship. Right now, we're thinking she will pursue a doctorate in American History.

I will continue working with Jonathan and Martha here at home. Although our priorities will be character development, they both do well academically. Jan had outlined a course of study for both of them. With all the experience we've had home schooling the older three, I expect we'll have no problems with the younger two.

As for me, the IMB is generous to give me up to a year to adjust to being a single parent and guide my kids through this transition time. So far, I'm still NED (no evidence of disease). Since mine was an aggressive cancer like Jan's, it would have likely reoccurred within three years of my surgery, which was in May of 2004. Otherwise, I now have good odds of staying cancer free, although a chance of reoccurrence remains possible for several more years.

If I stay healthy, I'll probably set my sights on returning to the Philippines sometime before Christmas. Jonathan and Martha would return with me. The Lord called me to missions before I met Jan, and I don't sense any change in the calling. The needs overseas are still enormous. There's still so much to do.

A few days after the Memorial Service, the children opened their first letter from Mom (written in the Fall of 2005). After writing individually to each one, Jan wrote these words to all:

I think back on my life and times when I was traveling or others in my family were traveling. You know, it's always easiest on the one who is on a trip, because there are new things for that person in store. It's hardest on the ones left at home, because life and routine must go on, and yet you feel the void left by the one that is gone. Like when David went to college; we were acutely aware of his absence. I never could figure out how many plates to set for lunch and I don't remember how long it was that I went to call him for meals – only to stop myself and be reminded that he wasn't there.

I guess it will be similar to my absence. It may be sometime before the "I'll go ask Mom" thoughts pass.

But you don't need to say, "I lost my mother on…". Nope. I am not lost – I had a destination when I left and we will see each other again! *"Tears of joy shall stream down their faces and I will lead them home with great care"* (Jeremiah 31:9). Because I am absent in the body means that I am at home with Jesus. I have always longed for a permanent home; now I have one!

Of course, I have no idea what you might be feeling at this time. But I hope that you are diligent to put on your daily armor of God (Ephesians 6) because Satan would love to use my homegoing to hurt you. And since so much of our battle with Satan takes place in our minds, it is so important for you to have right thoughts, thoughts that are according to God's Word which is TRUTH…

You may feel relief because I'm not battling cancer anymore and I've entered into my eternal reward. Relief can be a normal reaction. But if you feel this way, you may then also feel guilty because you don't feel so sad. (ARRGH! Emotions!) Don't let Satan try and condemn you ("You must not really love your mom or you would be sadder that she is dead"). It is okay to rejoice that I am in heaven. That doesn't mean that you love me any less…

You may feel denial, telling yourself, "it can't really be true. My mother isn't really dead. She will come back." Even though this is something that we have talked about for months and have known could happen, there can still be denial. Denial is a normal emotion… Give each other space to work through grief in your own way. Denial is usually temporary. It may come and go, but don't linger in it.

You may feel angry at the doctor, at the hospital, at some well-meaning visitor, even at God. Don't feel bad about being angry… You can always talk to God about how you feel. He can handle your anger. But you need to move out of anger… God is ready to pour out His grace on you to help you deal with the situation. Accept it. Rest in Him. Trust Him.

You may feel depressed. "Life isn't worth living. This is terrible." It's okay to cry; crying is a natural part of the grieving process. Jesus wept when He heard about his friend Lazarus's death. God promises to wipe away our tears (Revelation 7:17; 21:4). The Bible says to week with those who weep (Romans 12:15).

Hopefully, you will arrive at acceptance. You have worked through the above feelings of grief and can accept this as God's permissive will. Not only do most people go through these stages, but you may go through them and then still go back again and repeat some stages. (That can be frustrating when you think you have worked through it already!) It is OK if you are still grieving when other family members seemed to have moved on. Each person is unique and has their own time table.

Finally, no matter how wonderful heaven is, I would not choose to leave you to come here. There is nothing that you have done that would make me want to leave you. I love you very much. Neither is there anything that you have done that caused the cancer or made it worse. We live in a sinful world with lots of toxins and so there is disease.

But heaven is a glorious place. There is no more pain or suffering here. No tears. Death is ugly and it is repulsive but it is not able to bring the life of a Christian to a dreadful halt. I live on in the presence of my Savior! What a wonderful hope.

I love you. I am so glad that God allowed me to be your mother. Love, Mom

Words of Affirmation

In the weeks preceding Jan's promotion and in the weeks following, we received numerous notes and cards from people testifying of the impact Jan had on their lives. Here are some:

"My life will forever be changed. You have taught me more about our Jesus than you will ever know. You have displayed so many Godly characteristics. You have shared your faith with such grace and love. I stand amazed at the strength that God has given you."

"In all my years of ministry I have not seen such pure Faith and Trust in our Lord and Savior Jesus Christ. Your family has blessed us beyond all measure." (North Carolina)

"Her passionate love of people, flowing from her love of the Lord was stunning. She was resolved to do the will of God in ALL situations."

"She is a great example to me of how a Christian can be in any situation - firmly grounded, pressing on with a strong faith, generous, joyful, encouraging, seeking only to please her God. She is a treasure to a lot of people." (Philippines)

"She was so FUN to be with."

"She wanted her kids to know the Lord and love Him with all their hearts and nothing else was nearly as important as that. Every situation became an opportunity to learn about God. (Philippines)

"Sometimes when I felt defeated and overwhelmed she cheered me on giving me the confidence to continue." (Philippines)

"I only met her once but she inspired me SO much, with her strength, her courage, and most of all, her Faith! Even though she was in much pain at the dinner, she made a point to go to each person (approximately 30 of us), introduce herself, and ask how WE were doing!"

"I want to let you know that your family's testimony is pointing us and others to the sovereignty and sufficiency of God." (Missouri)

"Yours is the sweetest family I believe I have ever known."

"God has spoken to me through your family and your amazing faith. Words can't even describe how you have touched me and so many others."   (Missouri)

"I learned to love a fabulous family. Jan actually called my house one night when our circle was meeting and I think she talked to everyone! I can truthfully say I've never known anyone like Jan, so trusting, so full of grace and faith, and at the same time concerned about everyone else." (Georgia)

"In August I found out I had cancer, and laughed with joy as I knew why I had Jan as my mentor. I am having so much fun with my cancer, making people laugh and remember their faith... Thanks to Jan, I have the peace that passeth all understanding." (Indiana)

Jan carried a deep passion for Filipinos. She consistently asked for "how to pray" lists from friends and others. Her God-given passion is bearing fruit that remains." (Philippines)

 "I still remember the first time I met Jan. She was telling everyone at mission meeting of how their 4th child was born at home because they did not have time to get to the hospital. We laughed until our sides hurt. Nobody can tell a story quite like Jan."

"Thank you for modeling a life that is wholly sold out to the Lord - be it as a wife, a mother, a mentor, a friend - so caring, thoughtful, loving, full of fun and love for life. What an impact on those who have gotten to know you, myself included." (Philippines)

"My work and my life have been enriched through her inspiration and spirit." (Tennessee)

"I cannot think of Jan without smiling. She was joy. She was sunshine." (Virginia)

"You may not remember me, but I met you one day at [a doctor's office]. I just wanted to say that I was truly inspired by the faith you exhibited during the short time that we spoke and your conversations with others in the I.V. room. Your faith (in spite of serious medical problems) is truly inspirational."

"When I think of Jan, I think of the woman I want to be. She had something I respect and want in my own life, namely, order, grace, experience, wisdom, priorities, love, and fun. Jan, you made me a better missionary, mom, teacher, and disciple. Thank you!" (Philippines)

"Thank you for showing me my Savior."

"Of all the heroes on this earth, you are mine. Thank you for all that you have taught me through your testimony. Thank you for always giving our Lord and Savior Jesus Christ the glory in all things. You are amazing and if anyone on this earth understands what true selling out to the Lord means, I believe it is you." (Arizona)

"God is using your testimony in such a powerful way, to so many people! Thank you very much for your transparency that we may glimpse into more of who God is."

"Jan, through hearing you speak at our church, and through your journal, I have seen how strong your faith is in God. You have shown me there is hope and a reason why God uses such difficulties in our life so that the Lord will be honored and praised."

"I can see JESUS IN HER LIFE!" (Philippines)

"The radiance of Jan's countenance always spoke volumes to me. Psalm 34:5 often comes to mind when I think of her, "Those who look to Him are radiant and their faces are unashamed."

"Never have I met someone who demonstrates Christ as well as Jan." (Washington)

"Surely through her illness, Jan has touched many souls by her knowledge and application of God's Holy Word and made tremendous spiritual impact on many of us on our pilgrimage to our real home."

"I have cried, laughed, prayed and shared Jan's giant perspective of her God in her life. She has encouraged me and given me a new wonderment of the God that we serve."   (Florida)

"I only knew Jan for a few short months, and yet she touched my heart profoundly. She had such a peace about her. She shared with me the love she had for her children, the acceptance of her diagnosis, and how God's Word gave had given her strength. I drew such inspiration from her... Her faith was so unwavering. She was a rock of comfort, compassion, wisdom, and grace."

"I know it has blessed me to see her walk in the Grace of our Lord Jesus Christ, strong and steady with that sweet smile on her face. "

"The words that you left me with that day penetrated through my facade of extreme selfishness and pride. I thought, how can you have such peace in the midst of inevitable loss? Where does that unshakeable certainty in the infallibility of God's Word come from? I knew that God, Himself, made you for me for that very day. Through you, He restored to me my sense of purpose and value as His precious child."

"As we [a church in the Manila] read your letter, we see God actively working in your life. We continue to praise HIM for revealing Himself to us through your life. Your testimonies have touched and keep on touching lives. We have used your life testimonies to encourage the sick, the poor, and people who are so discouraged with their lives. We have seen over and over again that God can use even your illness for HIS GLORY."   (Philippines)

"Jan and you, Mark, have made such a difference in my life. I pray more and I believe more. I am hungrier for Our Lord and my life will never be the same after hearing from you two and your wonderful kiddos."

"Jan I have always had great respect for you and have always thought you are one of the greatest missionaries I have known in the Philippines. All of your life has had eternal significance. I am honored to know the great saint that you are. Thank you for being a powerful testimony to me of your great faith, and the way you have filled your mind with the Word of God throughout your life. Your lives have impacted my life for ever. I have been blessed!"   (Philippines)

"I love the glory of God that shines in your life. I love the way God has planted you as a mighty oak of righteousness that displays His glory. I just love you, my Yahweh sister."

"She was truly the most selfless and spiritually positive person I've ever known."   (Georgia)

"You are the one who recognized in the 90's it was time for the Central Philippines to fulfill its role of being a missionary sending region. God gave you the vision and faith that the people of that area... should now lead out in going and sending Filipino missionaries to unreached people groups. Many who you talked to about missions have now gotten the vision and are on the field or are leading churches to support those who are going."   (Philippines)

"We anticipate that the precious seed of Jan's life testimony sown in Chinese unbeliever's hearts will bear much fruit."   (Taiwan)

"The JOY of the Lord is indeed our strength and I see it in your example." (Philippines)

"Jan has been a living proof of a loving God to a watching world. The Lord has used her and her family to teach me about total surrender to the will of God, to teach me about prayer, to teach me about worship! The Lord has been glorified through her life. Every time I think about Jan and pray for her I get a little closer to Jesus."

"You are a treasure. There are more people on this earth who have been encouraged and bonded with you than anyone I know."

"You have had an eternal impact on people all over the world because of your love for and commitment to Jesus."

Words of Life

In Georgia, on Sunday, February 11, the day before Jan's Memorial Service, Gray Baptist Church celebrated their church anniversary. This is the church where Jan served while working for the U.S. Fish and Wildlife Service in 1980 and 1981. This is the church that, for many years, sent out our prayer letters. On this memorial Sunday, the pastor preached about the characteristics of the godly, verses that of the ungodly. He concluded his message with an illustration:

...Two women died last week. One was named Jan Moses. The other was named Vickie Lynn Hogan. Jan Moses loved the Lord and lived for God. Jan was a member of our church while working at the Piedmont National Wildlife Refuge. She came to church regularly; she wanted to be with God's people. While she was here, she sensed God's call to missions. So she resigned her position with the U.S. Government and moved to Texas to attend seminary. While there, she met Mark. They were married and appointed as missionaries by the International Mission Board. They spent years in the Philippines planting churches and helping people grow into those who glorify God.

She came back to the States after being diagnosed with cancer. Empowered by the Holy Spirit, she bore witness throughout her times of suffering of God's providence and plans for her life. Last week, she had a great homegoing. Tomorrow, they are going to have a celebration in which they will wear, not dark colored clothes, but light colored clothes, because they are celebrating her promotion into heaven with God.

The other lady who died was Vickie Lynn Hogan, also known as Anna Nicole Smith, a Playboy supermodel. On a TV spot about her life, a newscaster said, *"Her life was like a roadside wreck. Hard to watch, but difficult to ignore."* Possessing money, fame, and fortune, she once asked herself, *"Is this it; is this all there is?"* Mrs. Smith's life was ruthless, fruitless, and hopeless.

Now, how do you want your life to end? Like a Jan Moses, or like an Anna Nicole Smith? I am amazed that people say that I want to end like a Jan Moses, but live like an Anna Nicole Smith. How can you say that I want to arrive at the destination of the righteous, but live the lifestyle of the wicked? Friends, it doesn't work that way.

You and I must be among those who have the discipline of God's Word in our lives, who, on a daily basis, spend time in God's Word, reading it, hearing it, delighting in it, meditating on it, and applying it to our lives. So that when we arrive at the end of our days we can say, "I did what I was supposed to do and I arrived where I wanted to arrive, and I can hear the words of the Lord, Jesus Christ, saying, *"Well done, my good and faithful servant.'"*

What set Jan apart was not the love she had for people or the joy she had in life. These were the fruits of a deeper uniqueness – her passion to love God with all her heart and mind. And this passion found its most outward expression in her diligence to hide God's Word in her heart. As Jan would often say while holding her Bible, *"These are not mere words; they are my life!"*

It was these Words of Life that taught her to value what was eternal; to measure her days by how best she could express her love to God and share that love with those whom He brought into her life. It was these Words of Life, and her obedience to them, that made Jan into a beautiful lady with an uncommon faith.

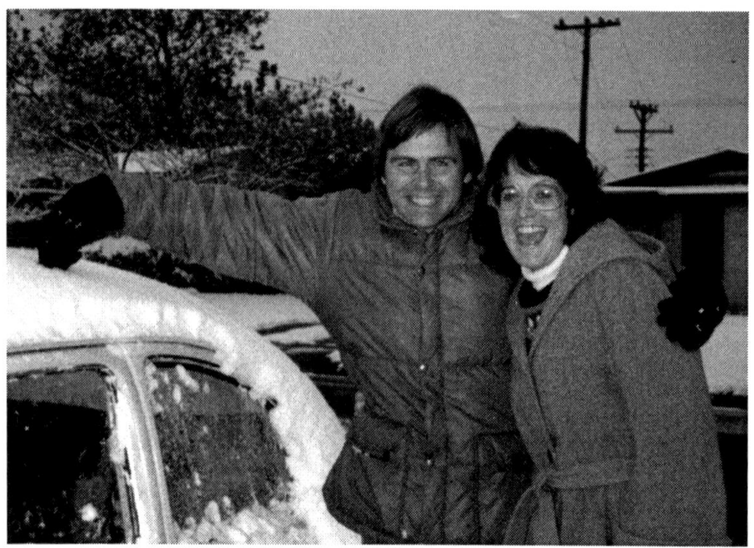

Mark and Jan - December, 1983

Appendix 1: God and Cancer

In March of 2004, my wife, Jan Moses, was diagnosed with melanoma, a very aggressive form of skin cancer. A surgery in April revealed lymph node involvement. The five-year survival rate for stage III melanoma is less than 50%.

On April 28, 2004, I was diagnosed with renal cell carcinoma, or kidney cancer. In May I had my left cancerous kidney removed along with two positive lymph nodes. The five-year survival rate for stage III kidney cancer is around 30%.

Although Jan and I have never asked the following question, we know some have: Why would a loving God allow a missionary couple in the prime of their ministry, with five dependent children, to both get cancer?

The answer is like a puzzle with many pieces. While Jan and I may never have all the pieces this side of heaven, God's Word provides us with enough pieces to form a clear picture that allows us to say, along with Job, *"Though He slay me, yet will I trust in Him"* (13:15).

Piece #1: GOD IS NOT RESPONSIBLE FOR MY SUFFERING

God's creation was perfect; there was no suffering. Hate, greed, immorality, sickness and disease came because of man's sin – his turning away from God. It will not do to blame God by saying He could have prevented Adam and Eve from sinning, for none of us would wantonly exchange our free will for robotic obedience. In addition, it is our sinfulness that reveals to us the true greatness of God's mercy; to see a holy God who lovingly and personally took my sin and died in my place so that He could have me live with Him in eternity.

God is not to be blamed for cancer. We, and all who came before us, are to be blamed. Our sin is to blame, along with all the viruses, toxins, and diseases that are part of God's curse on this planet because of sin (Genesis 3: 17-19). What is amazing is not the presence of suffering, but that a holy God would provide sinful people with a way out; a salvation for those who, by God's grace, continued to put the pieces together.

Piece #2: I DESERVE ETERNAL PUNISHMENT

The smallest sin is like a single cancer cell that renders the body diseased and unworthy of eternal perfection in heaven. Sin is a slap in the face of a holy God; a choice of rebellion that leaves me deserving of His most severe retribution. Sin is so serious that God pronounces death as its only justifiable payment. Doing good deeds, praying daily, serving 18 years as a missionary, or even living in perfection for a number of years (if that were possible), can never pay the penalty of death my sins deserve. Sin is that serious; God is that holy.

Therefore, whatever suffering I experience on earth is still far less than what my sins deserve. But oh, how grateful I am, that as an eight year old child I believed Jesus Christ paid my sin-penalty of death, and I rested in His promise that He would one day free me forever from all suffering.

Piece #3: THE CROSS IS MY EVIDENCE OF GOD'S LOVE

A few months ago I asked a Bible study group what was their evidence that God loved them. One said, *"He protects* me." Another said, *"He provides things for me."* Still another said, *"He gives me good health."*

I then asked if they thought God loved Job (the Old Testament sufferer). *"Of course,"* they replied. I then pointed out how God took away Job's protection, how God permitted his 'provisions' to be destroyed, and finally how God allowed Job's health to fail. But God still loved Job.

The lesson here is that we never measure God's love by our circumstances, for Satan can influence our circumstances to make us doubt God's love. But Satan can never take away the cross – the ultimate evidence of God's love. Paul, whose protection, provision, and health were diminished on many occasions said, *"May it never be that I should boast, except in the cross of our Lord Jesus Christ, through which the world has been crucified to me, and I to the world"* (Galatians 6:14).

For us cancer folks, we don't need healing to prove God's love. The cross is the only evidence we will ever need to be certain that God is for us, regardless of our circumstances.

Piece #4: MY HOPE IS IN HEAVEN, NOT IN HEALING

If God were to heal me of cancer, I certainly would not complain. But if he doesn't, then the nearness of heaven will be my comfort and joy. Whatever sadness I feel at leaving family, friends, and ministry on earth will be quickly erased the moment I behold the beauty of my eternal home. *"Things which eye has not seen and ear has not heard, and which have not entered the heart of man, all that God has prepared for those who love Him"* (1 Corinthians 2:9).

Piece #5: GOD'S WILL FOR ME ON EARTH IS HOLINESS

God has promised me eternal happiness in heaven. But on earth, *"all who live godly in Christ Jesus will suffer..."* (2 Tim.3:12). My purpose now is to *"live by faith."* *"For without faith it is impossible to please God"* (Hebrews 11:6). The greater my faith, the more God is pleased. And what better way to grow my faith than for Jan and I both to have cancer in the prime of our lives with our children still dependent on us!

If my faith grows and remains strong in the midst of such circumstances, then my cancer becomes a way for me to fulfill my purpose and calling in life. If a strong faith now will bring greater pleasure to God rather than lesser faith the rest of my life, then cancer is what I will choose. Sure, I want to serve the Lord as long as I can on earth. But my greater desire is to please my savior and Lord, Jesus Christ.

Piece #6: ONE OF GOD'S GREATEST PLEASURES IS GIVING

One of my greatest pleasures as a father is watching my children open their gifts from me on Christmas day. God says that it is *"His good pleasure to give you the kingdom"* (Luke 12:32). My first day in heaven will be like a child on Christmas Day, when my Father will reward me for my faithfulness here on earth.

These *"treasures in heaven"* will be greatly appreciated because I know I don't deserve a single one. It is only through the power of God's grace working in me that anything good comes from my life. But God *"is a rewarder"* (Hebrews 11:6) who gives rewards because it is His nature to do so, even if we don't deserve it. *"For God so loved the world that He gave..."*

My good works and years of missionary service add up to absolutely nothing in terms of my eternal destiny – heaven or hell. That is determined by my relationship to Jesus Christ. But my quality of life in heaven will be greatly affected by my faithfulness here, or lack of it.

Is it not rather easy to have faith when life goes well? But if God summons Jan and I to a higher faith by allowing both of us to have cancer, then shouldn't we see such a challenge as an opportunity to show our trust in Him? If such a level of faith will bring me greater treasures in heaven than a longer life with smaller steps of faith, then why would I want to pray for healing?

Of course, if God chooses to heal Jan or me or both of us, we will be glad and grateful. But if he doesn't, we know our faith will please God and bring us exciting rewards in heaven.

Piece #7: ABSENCE OF HEALING CAN BUILD ONES FAITH

Which requires a greater level of faith? To pray for healing and then be healed? Or to pray for healing and not be healed? If we base our faith on the observable evidence of an answered prayer, then it is no longer faith, because *"faith is the evidence of things we cannot see"* (Hebrews 11:1). I believe sometimes God may withhold our request in order to lead us to a higher level of trusting faith in Jesus Christ alone.

Piece #8: GOD MAKES CHOICES FOR MY ETERNAL BENEFIT

I would like to be healed of cancer so I can be the one to raise my children, to minister in the Philippines, to grow old with my wife. But all of these are rather selfish reasons.

Instead, I pray that God will be glorified through this cancer.   Healing is one way for God to be glorified, but there are others. For example, He may choose not to heal me so that...   1) my faith can be made stronger, 2) my rewards in heaven made greater, 3) my testimony might encourage others, 4) my rewards in heaven may not be lessened by possible wrong choices in the future, 5) my children may experience provisions I could never give them, and 6) many other ways that I can be benefited and He can be glorified through adversity.

For now, Jan and I will do all we can to get well. We desire healing, but our hope is in the Lord. If He should allow our cancers to return, to permit the curse of this world to take its course, then we will aim to show our trust in the Lord for however many days He gives us. If He should choose to heal us, whether through medicine or miracle, then we will continue to say, along with Paul, *"For me to live is Christ; to die is gain"* (Philippians 1:21).

And whenever I do stand before my Lord, on that Christmas-like day, I will have no regrets for the choices I have made: to leave home for missionary service; to sacrifice for my family; to remain faithful to my wife, before and after marriage; and to tell of God's love, whether in sickness or in health. And whatever pieces of the puzzle may still be lacking, I know He will supply them when I see Him face to face.

Appendix 2

A Faith Like Theirs Isn't Easy to Fathom by Steve Blow

I grew up in church hearing often about "peace that passeth understanding."

I always liked that phrase.

A more modern translation might be "peace that just flat-out boggles your mind."

I'm not sure I had ever really witnessed that kind of mind-boggling peace until a recent afternoon.

In Mesquite, of all places. While supper was on the stove.

I was a guest in the home of Mark and Jan Moses and their five children.

This is a family accustomed to foreign terrain. For almost 20 years, Mark and Jan have been Southern Baptist missionaries to the Philippines. The kids grew up there.

"It's kind of home to us," Jan said wistfully. And Mark added, *"We want to go back if at all possible."*

But first mark and Jan must deal with some even more unfamiliar territory.

Back in March, while still in the Philippines, Jan had some troubling skin spots removed. And soon she got bad news – melanoma, a very aggressive skin cancer.

A few weeks later, Mark had a troubling little event himself. *"I noticed blood in my urine and said, "Hey, that's not normal."*

One test led to another, and soon, Mark was given an almost unbelievable diagnosis – a cancerous kidney tumor.

In the span of about a month, the husband and wife were both diagnosed with life-threatening cancers.

"We have learned a lot about cancer!" Mark said with a laugh. And Jan chuckled, *"We sure have."*

And my mind boggled.

He's 46. She's 47. Both have cancers with less than a 50 percent survival rate after five years.

Yet Jan can laugh about Mark and his copycat cancer. *"I joked that he thought I was trying to get to heaven faster than him."*

Now, lest you think these people are just nuts, of course they have sad times. They want to see their children grow up.

Their eldest, 18-year old David, sat nearby as we talked.

Their next two, 16-year old Sara and 14-year old Hannah, were busy in the kitchen preparing dinner. Their youngest, 10-year old Martha and 8-year old Jonathan, were on their way home from day camp.

Years ago, Mark and Jan made a pact with another couple to raise the other's children should anything happen. That pact remains in place and has brought them great comfort.

Of course, Jan jokes, the friends made that pact when they had one child, not five. *"They are very committed to helping us get well at this point,"* she laughed.

Another tough part of this journey was leaving the Philippines so abruptly. *"Saying goodbye to everybody, not knowing if we will be able to go back – that was the hardest part,"* Mark said.

Mark and Jan said they have been humbled and awed by the outpouring of support for them. They left the Philippines with no idea of where they might live. *"And homes for a family of seven aren't the easiest to come by,"* Mark added.

Soon, Dallas' First Baptist Church made the spacious Mesquite home available to them. And though they were strangers to the church, members there have showered them with support.

"Sometimes I wonder if I could possibly be so kind to my friends," Jan confessed.

Of course, the question that always arises is one directed at God: "Why?"

But Mark and Jan said that question has never plagued them. *"We say, "Why not us? What's special about us?"* Mark said.

"For people who don't know the Lord; I know we sound odd or bizarre. But God never promised us we wouldn't have troubles.

"In fact, he promised us we would have troubles. But he also promises us he will always be there to walk with us through them."

"This is a bend in the road. A major, life-changing bend," Jan said with a smile. *"Things won't ever be the same. But all I can tell people is that God will walk us through it, and that's nice."*

That's nice?

No, that's a peace that passeth understanding.